Overcoming Incontinence

A Straightforward Guide to Your Options

MARY DIERICH, M.S.N., R.N., C-N.P.
FELECIA FROE, M.D.

John Wiley & Sons, Inc.

New York · Chichester · Weinheim · Brisbane · Singapore · Toronto

The information contained in this book is not intended to serve as a replacement for professional medical advice. Any use of the information in
this book is at the reader's discretion. The author and the publisher specifically disclaim any and all liability arising directly or indirectly from the use
or application of any information contained in this book. A health care professional should be consulted regarding your specific situation.

Library of Congress Cataloging-in-Publication Data:

Dierich, Mary.
    Overcoming incontinence: a straightforward guide to your options /
Mary Dierich, Felecia Froe.
        p.   cm.
    ISBN 0-471-34795-7 (pbk.)
    1. Urinary incontinence Popular works.   I. Froe, Felecia.
    II. Title.
    RC921.I5D54   2000
    616.6'3—dc21   99-36372
                                                                        CIP

Printed in the United States of America
10 9 8 7 6 5 4 3 2

CONTENTS

FOREWORD

For those patients suffering from incontinence, this book will come as a welcome relief. In spite of the fact that there are 17 million Americans who struggle with incontinence and that it costs our country 26 billion dollars annually, there are almost no books devoted to the topic. The adult diaper industry is a one-billion-dollar business. Incontinence is the number one reason for nursing home admission for the otherwise healthy elderly. It is not just a problem of the elderly, though, 20 percent of college coeds report episodic incontinence.

Incontinence can be prevented, is almost always treatable, and is often curable. Diapers needn't be necessary at both ends of our lives. For physicians who evaluate incontinent patients every week, this book is a welcomed adjunct to our practices. When I query my patients on what other information they would like, they invariably request something they can go home with, read, and share with their families. Excellent, well-written information on this topic has been difficult to find. That is why this book's contribution is so important.

What can you expect from *Overcoming Incontinence?* Mary Dierich and Felecia Froe have gained an expertise in the field of incontinence, and they offer the unique combination of both a nurse practitioner's approach and a physician's viewpoint. The definition of incontinence is thoughtfully discussed, and how and when to seek help is thoroughly covered. They take you through the steps of how incontinence is diagnosed and treated, what tests you might have performed, and what outcomes can be expected. They even spend a considerable length of time helping you navigate the maze of insurance reimbursement and HMO certification. Treatments are reviewed and the pros and cons of each debated. A well-informed patient is his or her own best advocate. Dierich and Froe will help you be just that.

As spokesperson for the National Association for Continence (NAFC), we applaud this effort to educate you the consumer. Incontinence robs people of their quality of life. We are looking to add life to years not just years to life. There is no dignity associated with incontinence. We treasure a well-written text for patients that can restore their dignity.

Lindsey A. Kerr, M.D.
National Spokesperson, National Association for Continence

PREFACE

Overcoming Incontinence takes you, the reader, through the reasons for bladder trouble, how you should normally urinate, and the red flags for problems that should be checked out. This book will help you pick a provider, help you get your care covered, and give you some hints to improve your situation before going to the doctor's office. After reading this book, you will feel comfortable speaking intelligently to your provider. Armed with this knowledge, you can participate in the decision making regarding your treatment. Finally, this book will empower you to take charge of your care. An informed consumer is a powerful consumer!

This book is for you if you

- have ever leaked urine
- had trouble making it to the bathroom
- feel that the way you toilet is "different"
- have had trouble with your back
- have had a difficult delivery of one of your children
- are approaching or are in menopause
- have had surgery on your back, abdomen, or pelvis

Readers are advised to seek the guidance of a licensed physician or health care professional before making changes in their health care regimens, since each individual case or need may vary. This book is intended for informational purposes only and is not for use as an alternative to appropriate medical care. While every effort has been made to ensure that the information is the most current available, new research findings, being released with increasing frequency, may invalidate some data.

ACKNOWLEDGMENTS

I am so grateful to . . .

My daughters, Sarah, Cynthia, Andrea, and Rebecca. Without their patience, constant encouragement, love, and help in running the house, this book would never have became a reality.

My husband, Anthony. The word *can't* is not in his vocabulary. Whenever an opportunity arises to try something new, he not only encourages me enthusiastically, he figures out a way for us to accomplish the job. I am blessed daily by his love and support.

And finally to the other men in my life, John Hulbert, M.D., and Randall Schapiro, M.D., mentors and friends. These gentlemen took a chance on an unknown practitioner and allowed me multiple opportunities to shine. Both not only believe in the contributions of nursing to medicine and consider nurses as colleagues, they never fail to acknowledge publicly the contribution of the nurses in their practices. They have always challenged me to think "outside the box" and to excel. Thank you.

Mary Dierich

To my husband Ian—always there, pushing me, encouraging me to be as good as I can be. Thanks, I love you. To my daughters, Takara and Reed—always there to remind me of what's really important. To the rest of my family—thanks for being there, always. To all of the urologists with whom I have worked—I have learned something from all of you. Thank you.

Felecia Froe

Introduction

*"The moment you alter your perception of yourself and
your future, both you and your future begin to change."*
—MARILEE ZDENEK

Urinary incontinence is the loss of bladder control or leakage of
urine that is a social or hygienic problem. This problem affects 15
percent of American adults at one time or another. Chronic incontinence especially affects women. It is estimated that one in four
women ages 30 to 59 has experienced an episode of urinary incontinence. At least 50 percent of nursing home residents are incontinent,
while 30 percent of all people over age 60 are incontinent. Medical
costs for treating incontinence and problems associated with incontinence, such as pressure sores and falls, total about $28 billion annu-
ally. Only a small percentage of this money (8 percent) is spent on di-
agnosing the problem. Adult absorbent products to contain urine
leakage cost $1.2 billion per year in the United States. Incontinence
is one of the major reasons cited for nursing home placement.

Unfortunately, too many people are suffering in silence and letting incontinence erode their quality of life. Have you been told that
little can be done about your incontinence? That it's simply a part of
growing older or a normal consequence of childbirth? Perhaps
you've never even discussed it with your doctor or anyone else. Only
30 percent of those bothered by incontinence actually mention it to
a health care provider. Often, they're ashamed or embarrassed, hid-
ing their problem from friends and family.

The good news is that incontinence is treatable in the vast majority of people. And, as you will learn in this book, there are more treatment options than ever before. Not only does *Overcoming Incontinence*

1

address the reasons for the bladder trouble you may be experiencing, but it presents many of the known ways to regain control, starting with the most conservative methods such as simple strategies and exercises, then explaining more involved treatments such as medications, incontinence devices, and surgery.

For each treatment option, we let you know about the benefits and risks. For instance, conservative treatments such as biofeedback and pelvic muscle stimulation require commitment to follow through. It may take weeks to correct the problem and a lifetime of exercises to remain successful, but conservative treatments generally are without side effects or significant complications. In contrast, surgery can immediately "fix" bladder problems, but not without risk. Postoperative care can be demanding, complications and side effects are possible, and the procedure may fail over time.

This book dispels the many myths associated with incontinence. It helps you find a caring, knowledgeable health care provider who will support and assist your treatment. It also gives you tips on getting insurance coverage for your care.

Incontinence: How It Starts and How to End It

Incontinence primarily affects women. It often starts insidiously with a drop or two of urine upon sneezing or coughing. Later, as menopause approaches, perhaps a pad will be needed to protect clothing during activities such as tennis, golf, or bowling. Soon afterward, running after a grandchild will be out of the question. As menopause passes, life begins to focus around how close the nearest bathroom may be, and finally, like a thief in the night, incontinence has stolen our dignity, freedom, and peace of mind.

Who Is Affected?

Although one in four women suffers with incontinence, that percentage does not change much throughout the life span. Incontinence can occur for many reasons. Urinary tract infections, vaginal infections or irritation, constipation, and certain medications may cause temporary incontinence. A variety of problems may cause permanent incontinence. Permanent incontinence often progresses from an initial problem of structural integrity to a problem of degenerative nerve changes, and finally to a problem of functional issues. Weakness of the bladder, the sphincter, or the muscles that support the bladder; overactive bladder muscles; a blocked urethra; neurologic disorders; or immobility can cause permanent incontinence. Anything that damages the nerves or muscles, such as back problems or neurologic diseases, can increase the risk of incontinence.

With problems such as dropping or prolapse of the bladder, uterus, or urethra, it is common that surgery is the only suggested course of treatment. Often, women believe that they should learn to manage the problem or are told that incontinence is a natural part of aging. These misconceptions are probably why only 30 percent of those bothered by incontinence actually mention the problem to a health care provider.

There are several types of incontinence:

• *Stress urinary incontinence* occurs when the pressure in the bladder exceeds the pressure in the urethra during times of increased intraabdominal pressure. This increased pressure usually occurs when coughing, laughing, sneezing, jumping, bending, lifting, or running. In severe cases, sometimes just walking or turning over in bed will cause leaking. As the name suggests, urine may escape during any activity that puts pressure or stress on the bladder even if the bladder isn't full. You may leak just a few drops or a stream of urine during these activities. In severe cases, you may lose urine continually. If you have stress incontinence you probably have given up certain activities that cause you to leak. You can usually predict pretty accurately when you will leak.

• *Urge incontinence* occurs when you can't hold your urine long enough to reach a toilet without leaking once the desire to void occurs. The phrase *overactive bladder* is often used to describe this condition. It may seem that you get no warning prior to the actual event. You might leak urine on the way to the bathroom, when turning the key in the lock trying to get into the house, when running water, or when stepping out into the cold. Sometimes the leak is just a squirt of urine, but more frequently, once the stream starts, it is almost impossible to stop. Generally, the leaking is very unpredictable. You can usually tell when someone has this problem because she may knock you over on the way to the bathroom.

• *Overflow incontinence* is the result of chronic urine retention in people who can't empty their bladder. Leakage occurs because the bladder has lost its ability to sense fullness or because the bladder opening is blocked. It can be blocked by an overfull rectum, an enlarged prostate, overactive pelvic muscles, or scar tissue formation from surgery. The inability to sense fullness is lost after prolonged overfilling of the bladder, nerve damage, or as a result of a disease such as diabetes or multiple sclerosis. The bladder continues to fill like a bucket under the faucet until capacity is reached and then it spills over. If you have overflow incontinence, you may have difficulty emptying your bladder and may push on your belly to start or maintain a flow of urine. Your stream is trickly or intermittent. At times, increased pressure may cause slight leaks of urine and sometimes you will leak continuously.

• *Functional incontinence* occurs in people who have mobility problems. You may have normal urinary control but can't get to the toilet in time because you are slowed by an injury, arthritis, stroke, or other physical or mental disorders. The disability may be permanent or temporary. Sometimes diseases such as Alzheimer's or depression can cause this problem. The drugs used to treat depression can make you sleep so deeply that you cannot wake up fast enough to make it to the bathroom quickly without leaking. People with Alzheimer's disease are often confused and disoriented upon waking and may need assistance to the bathroom, which may make it impossible to get there on time. When you have functional incontinence, you most probably will leak on the way to the bathroom, especially at night because less assistance may be available. It is not unusual to leak the entire contents of the bladder.

• *Iatrogenic incontinence* generally starts suddenly after changing medication dosage, being hospitalized, having surgery, or being restrained. For example, medication may have adverse effects on bladder function such as increasing frequency. Surgery may affect bladder function, either making the bladder more irritable or stopping its ability to contract at all for a few days. The excess fluids received through an IV may make it difficult for you to get to the bathroom quickly, especially if you are pulling an IV pole along. Hospital rails or restraints can make it impossible for you to get to the bathroom on time. If your situation or medications can be modified, the incontinence normally resolves.

As medical providers, we would be lucky if all incontinence were "pure," that is, only one type. However, most incontinence is *mixed incontinence*, meaning that the causes and the symptoms might overlap. If we solve one problem, another component may still exist.

Treatments Available

Many people with incontinence think their only options are absorbent products such as pads and undergarments. Until recently, most health care providers were quick to suggest surgery as the only course of treatment for structural problems such as dropping of the bladder, uterus, and urethra. However, twenty years of research evaluated in 1996 by the Agency for Health Care Policy and Research (AHCPR) has proven the efficacy of nonsurgical treatment. The AHCPR is a U.S. government–funded group of experts who composed a consensus guideline to be used as the foundation for treating incontinence. The guideline reviews assessment and treatment protocols and gives opinions on effective treatment for urinary incontinence. These guidelines are given only a passing nod by many health care providers and in many cases are ignored by Medicare, who, in effect, sets the standard for treatment by determining which treatments will be covered for payment.

Purpose of This Book

The purpose of this book is to dispel many of the myths of incontinence, to provide you with information about the options available, to inform you of the risks and benefits of each treatment option, and to help you to express to your health care provider your problem and its effects on your life, health, and happiness. In today's world, it is more important than ever that patients—and their health care providers—be well informed. We wrote this book because too many people think incontinence is inevitable or shameful. You have options. And no matter what the situation, an informed consumer is a powerful consumer.

> "We read books to find out who we are. What other people, real or imaginary, do and think and feel is an essential guide to our understanding of what ourselves are and may become."
> —Ursula K. LeGuin

ONE

Drip by Drip: How Our Plumbing Works

"An investment in knowledge always pays
the best interest."
—BENJAMIN FRANKLIN

The first step in overcoming incontinence is to understand how the body works; more to the point, how the urinary tract system functions. Knowing what is normal helps determine a course of treatment.

How the Urinary Tract Works

The urinary tract serves several purposes: producing urine, storing urine, and releasing urine in a timely manner. Urine is the liquid waste produced by your body and is made up of water, salts, and urea. Urine is made in the kidneys, which act as filters of the blood supply. The two kidneys produce urine at a rate of roughly one-half cup per hour. This rate stays constant unless affected by drugs or improved efficiency of your heart pumping blood through your system, such as when you lie flat or exercise. At any one time, the kidneys have one-eighth of the body's blood volume circulating through them (see Figures 1.1 and 1.2). Because the kidneys hold so much blood, they are very well protected by the body. The rib cage forms a protective bony layer over them and they are padded in a layer of fat.

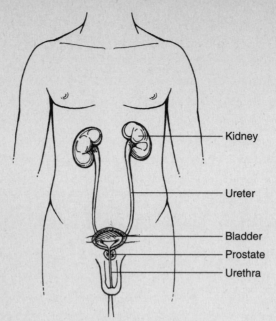

Figure 1.1. Front View of the Male Urinary System

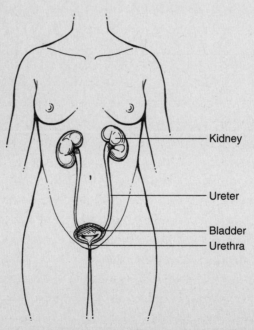

Figure 1.2. Front View of the Female Urinary System

Urine passes from each kidney through a narrow, long muscular tube called a ureter into the bladder (a hollow muscular organ), which acts as a storage container for the urine. The ureters connect under the bladder in a triangular area of specialized muscle called the trigone. The urine is moved along the ureters in half-tablespoon amounts by waves of contraction (peristalis) of the ureters. Normal urine is straw colored, clear, and without sediment. It can be darker if it is concentrated (more chemical waste products in a smaller amount of fluid), infected, has blood in it, or if you are taking certain medications. Urine is slightly acidic, which prevents bacteria from growing in the urinary tract. As the bladder fills, it stretches smoothly and passively at a low pressure. The bladder has stretch receptors that tell it when to stop stretching and start sending messages to the brain that it is filling. The bladder is sensitive to cold, irritants, and pressure, but little else makes it contract. When you are ready to pass urine, the pelvic muscle relaxes, the bladder contracts, and the urine flows through another larger muscular tube, called the urethra, and out of your body.

How the Urinary Tract Functions

The ureters, bladder, the internal spincter, and urethra are part of the involuntary set of muscles in your body—you can't consciously control the action of these muscles. Instead, they are controlled by a set of electrical impulses deep inside your brain, all without your awareness. This part of the brain controls the parasympathetic and sympathetic nervous system (the flight-or-fight system). These systems function in opposition to each other. If one system is active, the other system is not. Therefore, when you are under stress, one system is active and responding to chemicals produced by your body circulating in the bloodstream. When you are quiet, the other system is operative and different chemicals are circulating. The smooth muscles of your body—the stomach, bladder, and bowels—all respond to these circulating chemicals in a similar fashion—that is, by contracting faster when you are under stress.

In contrast, the pelvic muscles, which are connected from your pubic bone to your tailbone, are voluntary muscles, meaning you can control their actions by your thoughts much as you do your arm and leg muscles. However, when you are under stress, these muscles can also tighten, just like your neck and upper back muscles do. It is important to remember that these muscles are skeletal muscles, which means they can build up bulk just as you can bulk up your arm muscles by pumping iron. The pelvic muscles act as a sling to support the pelvic organs. These muscles wrap around the urethra, and in women look like a donut within a donut. Men have an additional structure, the prostate, which helps to maintain continence. The prostate gland is located at the junction of the bladder and the urethra. Its main purpose is to provide nutrients in the semen, which are needed for sperm survival. The pelvic muscles have two types of fibers: (1) fast fibers that react quickly and contract strongly and (2) slow twitch fibers that can sustain the contraction and hold the muscle in a contracted state for a long period of time. All these structures help maintain our bladder control. Although the kidneys are involved in urine production, they are not involved in the voluntary or involuntary loss of urine from the body.

The brain is also very intimately involved in our ability to control the bladder. The front part of the brain (the cerebral cortex) decides whether the time and place are appropriate for releasing urine while the back part of the brain (the pons) coordinates the bladder, urethra, and pelvic muscles to release the urine efficiently. In addition, the spinal cord provides the pathway for messages from the brain and bladder to travel back and forth. Indirectly, the prostate (in men) and the uterus (in women), as well as the pelvic bones and ligaments, supply support to the urinary tract and therefore affect its function. When surgery alters or removes these structures, the risk of incontinence increases.

How Voiding Occurs

The coordination of nerves, muscles, and thoughts is a truly beautiful process when everything is working properly. The kidneys make the urine, the bladder fills and stores the urine, and when full, it sends a message to the brain, saying, "I'm ready to go." If you are in an inappropriate place, such as in a meeting or the grocery store, your brain answers by signaling your pelvic muscles to tighten. When your pelvic muscles tighten, your bladder is signaled to stop squeezing (contracting) and to hold on a little longer. When you finally make it to the bathroom, your brain signals your pelvic muscles to relax, while it signals the bladder to squeeze, and like Niagara Falls, your urine is released (Figure 1.3).

Problems with Voiding

Although urinating may sound like a fairly simple process, and it certainly is not something you think about daily, it is in fact complicated

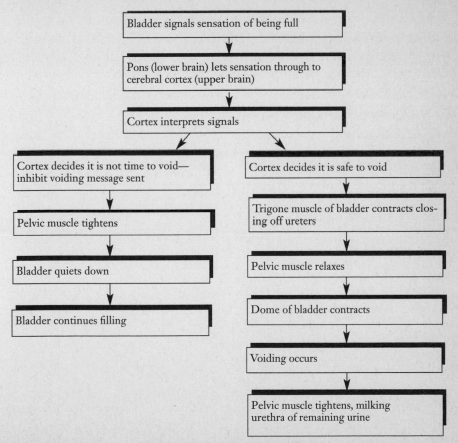

Figure 1.3. Steps in Voiding

and subject to pitfalls at any point or points along the way. Changes in the nerve pathways due to back injuries, stroke, or diseases such as multiple sclerosis can leave the muscles functioning abnormally. The pathway for the signals to operate the muscles (bladder, urethra, and pelvic muscles) are damaged and so the muscles can no longer do their job efficiently.

Surgery and childbirth can injure the muscles or nerves by overstretching and causing scar tissue both at the site of the surgery and near other organs. The muscles of the urethra and the pelvis then lose their ability to function well, although they are still receiving messages from the brain. Finally, diseases such as Alzheimer's can cause problems with the interpretation of signals sent to and from the bladder even though the nerves and muscles function properly. Several of these changes can occur in one person, so it is truly a miracle that we function as well as we do (Figures 1.4 and 1.5)!

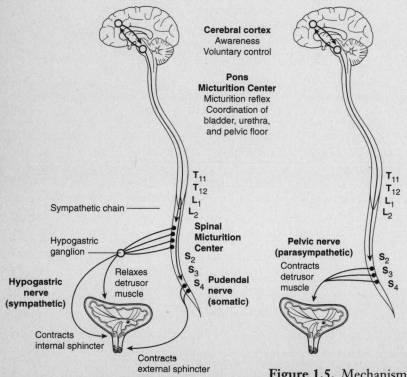

Figure 1.4. Mechanism of Continence

Figure 1.5. Mechanism of Micturition

TWO

What Happens When Our Plumbing No Longer Works

*"If you want to find the answers to the Big Questions
about your soul, you'd best begin with the Little Answers
about your body."*
—George Sheehan

Millions of people have bladder-control problems. There are four major types of incontinence. The first step toward successful treatment is determining the type of incontinence and the cause.

Stress Incontinence

Stress incontinence is the involuntary loss of urine that occurs with activities such as coughing, sneezing, and jumping. These are fairly vigorous activities, but some of you may also leak urine when just walking or turning over in bed. Stress incontinence occurs because the pressure in the bladder temporarily exceeds the urethral closure pressure during a maneuver that typically increases pressure in the abdomen. Many of you with this type of leakage have had children and have some degree of *prolapse* or dropping of your pelvic organs (bladder, urethra, or sometimes uterus).

One reason leakage with activity is thought to occur is because of weakness in the tissues supporting the bladder. This weakness allows

13

your bladder, more specifically your urethra, to drop below the pelvic floor muscles during activities. As a result, you leak urine. Sometimes damage to the back or tailbone injures the nerves coming out of the spinal cord, causing the muscles to weaken or not work at all. Although physically the muscles are capable of working perfectly, the message may not be received or the message is garbled. Diseases such as multiple sclerosis, spina bifida, or stroke can cause this problem. Compression of the nerves due to osteoporosis or repeated trauma to the spinal cord or tailbone can also cause this problem.

There are many women with prolapse of their urethra who do not have incontinence. Thus, many of us who treat incontinence believe that there must be another problem besides the fact that the organs have dropped. The pelvic floor muscles enter the picture at this point (Figures 2.1 and 2.2). By examination, we have found that many women with prolapse may not use their pelvic muscles correctly. Either they do not tighten them with strenuous activities or the muscles are so weakened that they no longer provide good support to the organs and allow the organs to move with activity. This movement causes the urethra to open when it should stay closed.

We also know that sometimes the muscles work correctly but are late in generating a contraction when needed with a strenuous maneuver. Other times, one side of the muscle works correctly, but the other side of the muscle does not move at all or moves sluggishly.

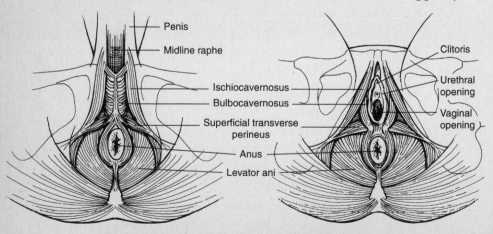

Figures 2.1. and 2.2. Muscles of the Pelvic Floor

Therefore, one side of the urethra is not closing well. The urethra may also not close efficiently due to lack of lubrication (creates a sticky mucous plug) or poor tissue "plumpness" (atrophy). Sometimes women bear down with lifting rather than tightening the pelvic muscles, further weakening the muscles. Some women just don't have a clue how to operate this muscle and relax it when asked to contract it.

To summarize, stress incontinence can occur for several reasons: weakening of the support tissues for the bladder and urethra, which result in prolapse; injury to the nerves that supply the urethra and pelvic muscles; and/or poorly functioning pelvic floor muscles. We will go into treatments for each of these problems a little later.

Probable Causes of Stress Incontinence

Weakness of the pelvic support muscles

- traumatic childbirth
- prolonged labors
- instrumented births
- being overweight
- chronic constipation and improper pelvic muscle use
- spinal cord trauma*
- neurologic diseases
- abdominal and vaginal surgeries

Poor closure of the urethra

- traumatic childbirth
- instrumental labors
- spinal cord trauma*
- neurologic diseases
- previous incontinence surgeries
- dilations of the urethra

*Spinal cord injuries include falls, nerve compression, disc problems, osteoporosis of the spine, as well as a broken back and whiplash.

Urge Incontinence

Urge incontinence is the loss of urine that occurs once you have the desire to go to the bathroom, but are unable to reach the facilities fast enough. This problem frequently occurs in conjunction with stress incontinence. Then the problem is labeled mixed incontinence. Often there may be urgency without the actual loss of urine. Many of you who have experienced urgency and/or urge incontinence on more than one occasion have begun going to the bathroom quite frequently to avoid the problem. This frequency/urgency syndrome is a vicious cycle. As you continue to go to the bathroom to prevent leaking, the bladder capacity becomes smaller and smaller, and you run to the bathroom even more frequently. The stream of urine becomes harder to start because there is not much urine in the bladder from the last time you went to the bathroom. The term *overactive bladder* has been coined to describe this condition. As with stress incontinence, there may be many causes for this problem. It may be due to changes in the nerves going to the bladder or to chemical irritants inside the bladder, or less commonly the cause may be a bladder neck that does not close completely. Examples of bladder irritants include highly concentrated urine, the chemicals released from bacteria during bladder infections, and substances that we might consume, such as alcohol, caffeine, or aspartame.

Changes to the nerves locally (in the pelvis) are usually caused by trauma or surgery. For example, an episiotomy done during childbirth may not heal well and may cause decreased or increased sensation of the pelvic area. A radical prostatectomy may cause the same problem. Central nerve damage (spinal cord trauma) not only causes some of the problems related to stress incontinence, but can also make the bladder more irritable, thus creating the feeling of the need to go to the bathroom more frequently.

The inside of the bladder, like the stomach, has a special lining that prevents irritants from attacking the bladder muscle itself. However, sometimes irritants are able to pass through this protective layer, usually during an infection or if the load of irritants is too much for the bladder to handle. There are also diseases in which this layer breaks down and leaves the bladder very vulnerable to chronic in-flammation. When the muscle becomes inflamed, it reacts to the ir-ritant by trying to get rid of it (contracting). Very concentrated urine can also cause this problem.

When the urethra does not close entirely, urine sits in the blad-der neck, which can make you feel as if you need to urinate all the time. Finally, running water, cold air, or trying to get into the house after being outside can provide a strong stimulus for the bladder.

Probable Causes of Urge Incontinence and Frequency

- poor habits
- infection
- poor closure of the urethra
- chemical irritants to bladder wall
- spinal cord trauma
- neurologic diseases
- local nerve damage
- not emptying the bladder completely

Overflow Incontinence

Overflow incontinence is due to an overly full bladder. It is different from urge incontinence because there is no urge to urinate when the leakage happens. An easy way to think of overflow incontinence is to think of a bucket under a running faucet that you forgot about. Eventually the bucket will fill to the top and overflow. This problem is common in men who have had longstanding prostate enlargement, though it does not happen to all men with prostate enlargement (Figure 2.3).

Other reasons that the bladder overfills include:

1. The bladder muscle does not contract efficiently enough to empty the bladder completely. This is common in diabetes, in multiple sclerosis, and with certain medications.
2. The sensation of needing to urinate is lost. This may happen

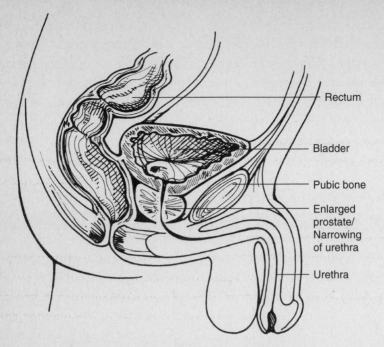

Figure 2.3. Urine flow with enlarged prostate

after a prostatectomy or as a result of a spinal cord injury or with diabetes.

3. There is a blockage of the urethra that prevents the bladder from emptying completely. This can happen with chronic constipation, scar tissue formation after surgery, and severe prolapse of the bladder, as well as with an enlarged prostate.

4. Pelvic muscles that don't relax properly.

The easiest problem to deal with is the blockage of the urethra. If blockage of the urethra is the cause of the incontinence, it is removed or reduced. If the blockage is due to the prostate, it can be partially removed surgically or treated with medications that help it to relax. If you remove the blockage, the bladder should be able to function again. However, chronic overfilling can cause permanent changes in the bladder wall, for example, in men with enlarged prostates. Notice the above picture of the male urinary tract with the prostate at the opening to the bladder. As your prostate enlarges, your bladder must work harder to empty. At first, your bladder muscle becomes stronger and thicker, but over time it may decompensate and become unable to squeeze to empty well, like an overstretched balloon.

If scar tissue is the problem, it must be reduced surgically. Often, none of these are the case and we find that the problem is overactive pelvic muscles. This can be treated with medication (muscle relaxants) or muscle retraining (as with biofeedback).

Other causes of this problem are diseases such as diabetes or multiple sclerosis. As we learned previously, the nerves that signal the bladder to contract and the nerves from the bladder that signal fullness no longer deliver their messages to and from the brain and the bladder. Without signals, the bladder just keeps filling.

Three common situations can cause overflow incontinence. It can occur when you cannot relax the pelvic muscles completely and the bladder has to work harder to empty, like the bladder in prostate enlargement. Women who have severe prolapse of the bladder commonly have trouble emptying their bladder because urine becomes trapped in the part of the bladder that has dropped. Finally, people who have trauma or surgery on the urethra can form a stricture (narrowing of the channel) of the urethra that prevents the bladder from emptying completely.

Probable Causes of Overflow Incontinence

Poorly contracting bladder

- chronic bladder overfilling because the toilet is not convenient, for example, flight attendants, nurses, surgeons, teachers
- neurologic diseases
- spinal cord injuries
- diabetes
- Parkinson's disease

Occlusion of the urethra

- prostate enlargement
- chronic constipation
- inability to relax pelvic muscles

continued

- severe prolapse of the bladder
- Parkinson's disease, multiple sclerosis

Functional Incontinence

Functional incontinence is the last major problem seen in people who leak urine. Most people have about two minutes after they get to absolute fullness before the bladder starts contracting so strongly that they could leak urine. You may have functional incontinence after you break your leg or hip and can't get around as well as you used to. A disability may prevent you from getting to the bathroom on time. Clothing that is difficult to remove or distance to the bathroom or a restraint may prevent you from getting to the bathroom efficiently. The hallmark of this type of problem is usually incontinence on the way to the bathroom, usually of a large volume of urine, after sleeping through the night. Trying to wake up, getting out of bed, and getting to the bathroom on time is the problem rather than a poorly functioning system. People with functional incontinence may be dry during the day because they can plan their trips to the bathroom.

This problem may also be the diagnosis in people with psychologic or psychiatric disorders, such as depression or Alzheimer's disease. In these cases, the muscles and the nerves of the urinary tract function normally, but you can't get to the bathroom quickly enough because the portion of your brain that processes the signals from your bladder and then responds to them is not functioning correctly either because of the disease or due to the influence of drugs taken to combat depression or psychosis.

Probable Causes of Functional Incontinence

Changed ability to perceive the need to urinate

- medications that treat sleep disorders, anxiety, depression, seizures or psychosis
- narcotics to treat pain
- Alzheimer's disease and dementia

continued

People who can't get to the bathroom because of mobility problems

- arthritis of knees and hips
- joint replacements
- being confined to wheelchairs or beds
- neurologic disease
- physical restraints (used in nursing homes, hospitals)

Overlapping Types of Incontinence

As convenient as it is to neatly classify the four types of incontinence, some people have more than one type (Figure 2.4). You may have accidents in which you have a strong urge to void, but cannot reach the bathroom on time, for instance, if you have broken your leg and therefore can't get around as easily. The pain medication you might be taking for your leg may make you less aware of filling because it makes you slightly more sleepy. Thus, the urge to void is not felt in time to get to the bathroom. In addition, you might have problems

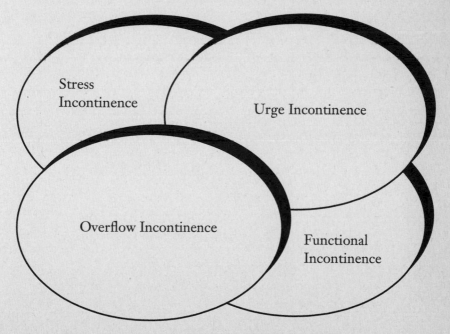

Figure 2.4. The Overlapping Nature of Incontinence

with accidents during activities that cause increased abdominal pressure, such as sneezing or coughing, because you are getting close to menopause. Perhaps, you might not be emptying your bladder completely because of bladder prolapse. The pain medications for your leg might make this situation worse because the bladder is not emptying efficiently due to the action of the medication. Although it might be easy to call this functional incontinence, it is clear that iatrogenic incontinence, overflow incontinence, urge incontinence, and stress incontinence also exist. If you had never broken your leg, you might never have been incontinent at all. However, the effect of the broken leg and the medication has set up a chain of events in which one problem worsens another. Treatment will require blending of modalities.

Now that you know the reasons for incontinence, let's examine some of the simple things you can do to improve your problem.

THREE

Starting from the Basics: What You Can Do Before Seeing the Doctor

"First say to yourself what you would be; and then do
what you have to do."
—EPICTETUS

There are simple things that you can check or do before making your first doctor's appointment. Changing some habits may improve your incontinence and save you the trip to the health care provider's office!

Diary Keeping

Before you even begin thinking about what kinds of things might be contributing to your problem, you must have an idea of when you are leaking, how often you are leaking, how much you are leaking, and what situations are associated with leaking. A simple diary is the easiest way to get at this information without a lot of work (Figure 3.1). If you end up going to your health care provider's office, the diary you've kept will be the most important information the provider will obtain about your patterns of leaking. When the provider can look at your patterns, the decision of how to treat your problem is more easily made. In addition, a diary will help you figure out which of your habits are preventing you from attaining continence (Figure 3.1).

23

Time	Fluid Intake	Urge to Toilet	Voided in Toilet	Number of Leaks	Changed Pad	Activity
6–8 A.M.						
8–10 A.M.						
10–Noon						
Noon–2 P.M.						
2–4 P.M.						
4–6 P.M.						
6–8 P.M.						
8–10 P.M.						
10 P.M. – Midnight						
Midnight – 2 A.M.						
2–4 A.M.						
4-6 A.M.						

Figure 3.1. Example of a Blank Diary Page

As you prepare to do your diary, select three days in a row that best represent your normal activities and fluid consumption (avoid vacations, new routines, etc.). Do not do your diary during your menstrual period. Going to the bathroom more frequently and more leaking is very common the week right before your period and during the first few days of your period. Using pads during your period will also change the pad count. It is essential to keep a full 24-hour record for each day.

Completing a Diary

In the first column, record the type and the amount of fluid you consume. This helps you to see which fluids may be detrimental to bladder control and whether you are drinking too little or too much. Keeping track of how much you drink is often the most difficult aspect of keeping a diary. It may help you to measure two or three of your favorite glasses to see how many ounces they hold. Then while keeping your diary, use just those glasses. The measurement does not have to be exact, but it should be a close estimate. In the next column, make a check every time you think you need to go to the bathroom (for instance, when you are shopping and the rest rooms are on the other side of the mall)—that is, you've received a signal from your bladder making you aware that you may need to go soon. In the third column, make a check each time you use a toilet to empty your bladder.

Sometimes you might leak before you get to a toilet. If so, make a check in the fourth column each time it occurs during a given time period. In the next column, make a check each time you put on a new pad. If you use different-size pads or diapers during the day than at night, make sure to designate which size you use. The final column is to help you remember what you were doing when leakage occurred. Sometimes, you may not know when you leak, so you won't be able to fill in the column. That's significant, too. Just be sure to tell your health care provider the reason the column is not complete. As you can see, the diary can give you quite a bit of information (Figure 3.2).

Fluid Factors

People with bladder problems all too often limit the amount of fluids they consume, thinking that the more they drink, the more they'll leak. The problem is, drinking less than the ideal amount (normally six to eight 8-ounce glasses of fluid per day) causes the urine to be so concentrated that the bladder contracts more frequently to eliminate the irritating urine. Urine that is dark orange/yellow or has a strong odor is usually too concentrated. Although drinking more fluid will change the color to a straw color and decrease the odor, if you are

Time	Fluid Intake	Urge to Toilet	Voided in Toilet	Number of Leaks	Changed Pad	Activity
6–8 A.M.	1 c. OJ ½ c. Milk	Strong x1	√		√	Getting Dressed
8–10 A.M.						Working at desk
10–Noon	12 oz. H_2O		√			↓
Noon–2 P.M.		Strong x1	√			Out in Garden
2–4 P.M.	1 can soda (caffeine)			√√	√	↓
4–6 P.M.	1 Glass Milk	√				Making Supper
6–8 P.M.	2 Glasses Water		√			Watching T.V.
8–10 P.M.	½ c. H_2O	√	√		√	↓
10 P.M. – Midnight						Sleep
Midnight – 2 A.M.						
2–4 A.M.		√	√	√		
4-6 A.M.						↓

Figure 3.2. Example of a Filled-in Diary Page

drinking more than six to eight 8-ounce glasses of fluids per day, you may be drinking too much, increasing your frequency. Many people think that you will leak more if you drink more fluids. You will probably go to the bathroom more; however, if leaking is going to occur, it will happen no matter how much you drink.

The type of fluids you drink will also have an impact on how often you are leaking. If you enjoy caffeinated coffee, you better have a clear path to the bathroom! Caffeine changes the way your bladder works for a number of reasons. All the hollow organs that squeeze/contract (your heart, stomach, intestines, and bladder) have a special group of cells called pacemaking cells that determine how often the organ contracts. Caffeine is a chemical that increases how fast the pacemaker conducts its business. Therefore, when a person drinks lots of caffeine, whether it is in coffee, soda, or tea, the bladder will contract more frequently and more forcefully. This translates into a strong urge to go to the toilet. If the muscles controlling the opening to your bladder (the pelvic muscles) are weak, the bladder can contract with more force than your muscles can hold back and leaking occurs!

Caffeine also acts as a bladder wall irritant, much like concentrated urine, alcohol, and the artificial sweetener, aspartame, which is marketed as Nutrasweet and Equal. When these chemicals come into contact with the bladder wall, the bladder responds by trying to get rid of them (contracting). Like alcohol, caffeine is a diuretic, a chemical that makes the kidneys process urine more quickly. More urine made means more urine to be eliminated!

Therefore, one of the easiest changes you can make is to eliminate or decrease caffeine, alcohol, and aspartame intake as much as possible. An easy way to decrease caffeine consumption is to mix half decaffeinated coffee and half regular coffee. Another easy way to decrease caffeine intake is to switch to tea. While an 8-ounce cup of coffee has 240 milligrams of caffeine, the same amount of tea only contains 60 milligrams. Switching to herbal tea eliminates caffeine entirely.

Eliminating aspartame, particularly if you are dieting or diabetic, is more difficult. Any health care provider will tell you that water is the best fluid you can drink. Fruit juices, Kool-aid, and milk usually do not bother the bladder. However, an overdose of citrus fruits, citrus drinks, or vitamin C can irritate an already irritable bladder. One or two helpings of citrus per day are plenty, as is 1,000 milligrams of vitamin C (if you are trying to acidify your urine to prevent bladder infections).

Habits

Examining how often you have an urge to toilet and how often you actually toilet can lend some perspective to whether you are in the habit of toileting too frequently or really going when necessary (Figure 3.3). People who toilet for every urge they feel may benefit from a technique called urge inhibition that we will discuss more fully later in this chapter. Another way to stretch the capacity of your bladder is to use a voiding schedule. Look at the shortest amount of time between toileting episodes and try to go at least that long between toileting episodes for one week. The next week, try increasing the interval by five minutes. The following week, increase the interval by another five minutes until you can comfortably go three to four hours between toileting episodes. Naturally, it takes a long time to get to this mark if you started out going to the bathroom every half hour. One way to get to this point more rapidly is to use your pelvic muscles to help "hold" your urine (Chapter Seven) or to use medication to quiet the bladder (Chapter Six).

Coping with Urgency

The feeling of needing to go to the bathroom immediately or leaking on the way to the bathroom is urgency. Urgency can be caused by scarring of the bladder from radiation, surgery, repeated infection, a urinary tract infection, stones in the bladder, constipation, concentrated urine, polyps, cancer, neurologic diseases, a small-capacity bladder or a bladder that doesn't stretch easily to accommodate urine, diuretics, a dry or poorly estrogenized urethra, or substances that irritate the bladder wall. Bladder cancer is rare and usually presents with blood in the urine, which is picked up by a urine test called a urinalysis. Infection can be picked up by culturing the urine to grow bacteria, which is a very simple test. Both of these tests require only a urine sample. If crystals are seen in the urine when looking at a sample under a microscope, the urologist may look into the bladder to determine if there are stones. Probably the most common reason for urgency is that we get into poor habits to prevent leaking large amounts of urine. Eventually our bladders get used to holding smaller and smaller amounts of urine.

What Are Some Things I Can Do to Control Urgency?

The easiest and first thing to do is to eliminate chemicals that irritate the bladder and cause it to contract more frequently. These chemicals include caffeine, alcohol, citrus, carbonated beverages, and aspartame. One helping of these substances is okay; however, it is best to eliminate them from your diet if possible. Increasing fluids so that you are drinking six to eight 8-ounce glasses of fluid a day will dilute the urine so that it doesn't become an irritant to the bladder wall. In addition, good urine production flushes germs out of the bladder. It is important to drink plenty of liquid after intercourse if you are a woman prone to infections so that you will urinate a good volume within two or three hours after intercourse. Also, remember to wipe from front to back after using the toilet so that you do not bring bacteria from your anus to your urethra.

How Do I Find Out How Much My Bladder Holds?

Remember that the kidney normally produces about a half cup of urine an hour and almost everybody has at least this bladder capacity. Try measuring your urine output after sleeping for the longest period at night. This will give you a good idea of how much urine your bladder is capable of holding. For example, if your bladder holds 1½ cups of urine at night, your goal during the daytime should be three hours between toileting. Try to increase the time you hold your urine by five minutes every few days. Keep in mind that caffeine and alcohol make your kidneys produce urine at almost twice the rate they normally do. So if you continue to drink these fluids, you need to account for this. The way your health care provider finds out how much your bladder holds is by doing a simple test called a cystometrogram (CMG) in which a small tube (catheter) is inserted into the bladder through the urethra and fluid is put into the bladder until it is full or you leak. This test takes about a half hour and there is no preparation.

Is There Anything Else I Can Do?

Sometimes putting your feet up above the level of your heart before bedtime causes your kidneys to work more efficiently before you go to bed. This especially helps if you have heart problems or if you are on your feet a lot during the day. Sit in a recliner or put your feet up on some pillows or on the arm of your couch while lying down for 30 to 45 minutes before bedtime. Then right before bedtime, go to the toilet. This will increase the length of time you sleep without interruption.

We usually get only a two-minute warning before we leak if our bladder is at capacity. Therefore, if it takes you more than two minutes to reach the bathroom because of distance, heavy sleeping, or a disability, you have two choices. You can either get to the bathroom before your bladder reaches capacity or you can move the toilet closer to you by using a urinal or a commode. If your pants are difficult to unbuckle, switch to a snap opening or a Velcro fastener. Decrease the amount of medications that make you sleepy or set an alarm to wake you before your bladder reaches capacity. Put yourself on a two- to three-hour schedule of going to the bathroom. All of these things won't change the reason you are leaking, but they may improve your situation.

The chemicals made by your body during stressful situations can make your bladder contract more often. These chemical messengers are the way various organ systems within your body communicate with each other. An imbalance of these messengers can adversely affect the way an organ functions. If you recognize this and eliminate stress, chances are your toileting patterns will begin to normalize. If you are nervous about getting to the bathroom on time, your bladder will contract more often. The key to getting to the bathroom without

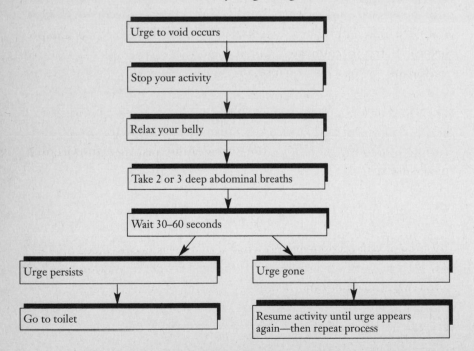

Figure 3.3. Urge Inhibition Strategy

leaking is to stop your activity when you get a strong urge, relax your belly (to take the pressure off your bladder), take a deep breath or two, and wait a moment until the strongest urge passes. Then walk to the bathroom since running jostles the bladder. If your pelvic muscles are strong and you know how to do a pelvic muscle contraction, use the reflex between the pelvic muscle and the bladder to calm the bladder down while waiting for the urge to pass. Do two or three quick contractions to signal the bladder that the "door out" is closed. Once the bladder gets this message, it will stop or slow its contractions.

As you get better at this procedure, if the urge has passed, continue your activity. Repeat this cycle until the urge can no longer be suppressed. At this point, you should respond to the urge and go to the toilet. Within about three weeks, you will notice that you can go significantly longer before needing to go to the bathroom.

What If These Measures Don't Help?

Your health care provider will probably try medication (see Chapter Six) or a machine called a pelvic muscle stimulator (see Chapter Seven) to try to calm an irritable bladder. If a woman is close to menopause or past menopause and her estrogen level is low, adding estrogen cream to the vagina can help lubricate the urethra and increase the tissue plumpness around the urethra. Frequently, further testing will be recommended to determine the cause of the urgency. Although incontinence is not life-threatening, testing is important to make sure that the incontinence is treated correctly.

Kegel Control

Looking at when you leak and what activity was taking place may also help you when figuring out some lifestyle issues to modify. Leaking with coughing, sneezing, bending, or lifting is usually related to poor pelvic muscle tone. Working on strengthening the pelvic muscles through exercise (Kegel muscle contractions) may help you regain control. In order for the exercises to be beneficial, they must be done properly (Figure 3.4).

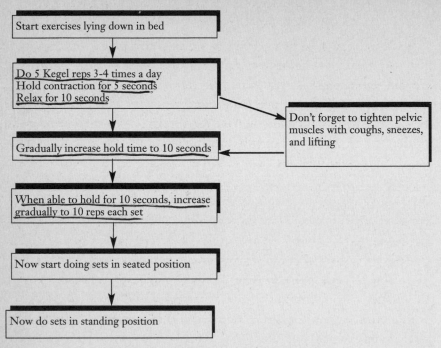

Figure 3.4. Kegel Exercise Progression

Strengthening the pelvic muscles is an important part of any continence maintenance program. You are never too old to strengthen these muscles. Damage to the pelvic muscles over time can be the result of precipitous, prolonged, or instrumented childbirths, tears or large episiotomies during childbirth, surgical procedures to the abdomen or pelvic area, injuries to the tailbone or spinal cord, neurologic diseases, chronic constipation, or decreased estrogen levels. If these muscles become damaged, the support for the bladder, rectum, and uterus changes. With decreased support, the bladder can open slightly with increases in abdominal pressure or the urethra can prolapse (drop). With surgical procedures, the urethra can scar in an open position. In addition, when the uterus is poorly supported, it can put pressure on the bladder, and if the urethra (the opening to the bladder) stays open, it can feel like you need to go to the bathroom even with very little urine in the bladder. The pelvic muscles can help you control the feeling of urgency and prevent leaking on the way to the bathroom.

How Do I Find the Pelvic Muscles?

The easiest way to activate these muscles is to think about the times that you have had the urge to pass gas in a public place. In order to prevent embarrassing yourself you tightened your anal sphincter muscle. Now, close your eyes and pretend you are in the elevator with the queen of England and you have terrible gas. Normally, you would tighten the anus (the opening from which stool passes). You are tightening the pelvic muscles. These same muscles need to be exercised regularly to prevent incontinence. Try not to use your legs, stomach muscles, or muscles of the buttocks. Another way to find these muscles is to try to stop or slow the stream of urine when you are urinating. However, don't do this too often (no more than one or two times a week) because you could learn some bad habits, such as no longer being able to relax these muscles. This would result in a urine stream that comes out in spurts and possibly you would be unable to completely empty your bladder. Some women visualize lifting or pulling up the muscles surrounding the opening of the vagina. If you place your finger just inside the vagina when you tighten these muscles, you can feel them tightening. A man can feel these muscles tightening by placing his fingertips on the skin just behind the scrotum. As the muscles tighten, you will feel them slide under your fingertips.

Remember from Chapter One that the pelvic muscles act like a hammock supporting the pelvic organs, but that they also act as a sphincter, a circular muscle that closes an opening from an organ. In order to make the muscle work most effectively, it must be used daily and exercised regularly. As this muscle does not move a joint, no one should be able to tell when you are doing a Kegel contraction. Your body shouldn't shift in the chair when doing this exercise, nor should your other muscles tighten. If you are having trouble, seek the help of a health care provider who specializes in treating incontinence to help you learn how to use this muscle correctly.

What Should I Expect?

If your pelvic muscles have been damaged, it will take some time to strengthen them. If you have broken your arm or leg, you know how shriveled the muscle looks after the cast is taken off. If you think of your pelvic muscle in a similar fashion, you will understand why it takes 12 to 16 weeks to rehabilitate. Don't despair. It took a long time to get to the point of leaking. With daily exercise, you will begin to notice less leaking in 4 to 6 weeks, although this improvement will not be consistent. As you begin to repair the muscle, it grows larger and the nerve density to the muscle must increase, causing the muscle to react faster when recruited with coughing, sneezing, and so forth. By exercising this muscle, you also increase the blood flow to it and squeeze the glands that lubricate the urethra. Increased lubrication helps provide a mucus plug to seal the urethra. Finally, during the last 6 to 8 weeks of daily exercise, the muscle begins to increase in bulk, just as your arm or leg muscles do when you lift weights. This increase in bulk helps to squeeze the urethra closed even when you aren't thinking about it.

Holding the contraction (an isotonic contraction) is the key to making the muscle sufficiently thick or bulky to help with passive urethral closure (putting the squeeze on the opening to the bladder). A thick muscle will help the urethra stay closed even when you aren't thinking about your bladder. A strong muscle, on the other hand, can be summoned into action quickly when the need arises, for example, when the bathroom is half a block away or you need to unlock the house after the car is parked in the garage.

How Many Exercises Should I Do?

The best way to determine how many exercises should be done is by using a biofeedback machine that measures the strength and the quickness of the muscle contraction during coughing and bearing down. An alternative would be to have a trained therapist feel the muscles when you are contracting them and time how long you can hold a contraction. If neither of these alternatives is available to you, try doing an exercise and holding the contraction for 10 seconds. If you can't hold the contraction for a full 10 seconds or you use your stomach, leg, or buttocks muscles, then only hold it for as long as you comfortably can. If you can hold a contraction for 10 seconds, then repeat it 10 times. Again, if you find yourself using muscles other than the pelvic muscle, it is time to stop. Be sure to rest between each contraction for 10 seconds.

Most people who are incontinent cannot hold a full 10-second contraction when first starting the exercises. They probably can't do more than three to five repetitions at a time. A safe starting point is three to five contractions three to four times a day. A good schedule is to do a set before you get out of bed, one set at noon, one at dinner time, and one before bedtime. Every few days, increase the hold time by one second, and once you can hold the contraction for 10 seconds, increase the number of contractions by one each set every few days until you get to 10 contractions per set. Initially, because the pelvic muscle is quite weak, you might not be able to exercise it easily when sitting up, because gravity is pulling against your efforts. If that happens, do your exercises when you are lying down or before you get up or go to sleep.

Can These Exercises Hurt Me?

If you get a little too enthusiastic about doing the exercises, you may find yourself leaking a little more. Like all muscles, if you overuse the pelvic muscle without conditioning it, you can overtire it. You may notice that leaking is worse toward late afternoon or early evening. Again, this is because the muscle gets tired by the end of the day. Be patient and continue to work at the exercises. You will be amazed at the results. However, remember, like other exercises, if you don't do the work, you won't improve.

Relaxation Is Important

Another reason people leak is because they don't give themselves enough time to empty completely. Leaking also happens when you ignore the urge to have a bowel movement. Eventually, you will become constipated. Constipation can cause urinary urgency, because the full bowel is pressing on the bladder. In very severe cases, it can obstruct the bladder neck so that the bladder can't empty fully and sometimes not at all! Obviously, this is a medical emergency. One of the best things you can do before going to the doctor is to make sure you are having an adequate bowel movement every day.

Make sure you are eating five to eight helpings of fruits and vegetables daily and drinking the right amount of fluids.

Relaxing completely in a busy world is difficult at best. However, it is crucial if you want to empty your bladder completely. If you find your stream is trickling, stopping and starting, or you have difficulty starting your stream, you may not be emptying completely. If this is happening despite your best efforts at relaxing, let your health provider know. You may have other problems that need medical attention.

Simple Steps to Try

There are many things you can do to prevent leaking:

- Think about how much fluid you are drinking. Six to eight 8-ounce glasses are sufficient for most days.
- Modify the types of fluids you drink. Water is always the best choice.
- Eliminate the "preventive" toileting. Help your bladder to hold more.
- Do a Kegel contraction with coughing, sneezing, lifting, and before taking off to the bathroom.
- Practice a Kegel exercise program faithfully.
- Eat five to eight helpings of fruit and vegetables daily.
- Relax completely when on the toilet. Forget the stresses in your life.
- Try to avoid sleep medications. Use meditation or relaxation techniques to help you get to sleep.

When incontinence does not resolve with simple lifestyle changes, it could be a symptom of a more serious medical problem, such as infection, diabetes, or neurologic disorders. It is always best to have incontinence problems checked by a professional, rather than letting a serious medical problem continue undetected. In the next chapter, you will learn how to deal with your insurance coverage.

FOUR

Getting the Care You Need: Speaking the Lingo

*"When the time for action has arrived,
stop thinking and go in."*
—Napoleon Bonaparte

Acknowledge That There Is a Problem

Once you've made the decision to seek care for your incontinence, how do you go about choosing a health care provider, and more importantly, how do you find one with whom you feel comfortable? Many health care providers do not ask women about this problem during their routine physicals. While women often assume that incontinence is the result of aging or childbirth, men view incontinence as abnormal and will mention it early in a discussion with their health care provider. It is up to you to raise the issue with your health care provider. You must convince your primary provider that this is a serious problem for you and that you want treatment. Medicine is rapidly changing in all fields and it may be that your provider is not aware of the newer conservative treatments for incontinence.

Choose a Provider

You may need to help your primary provider by giving him or her information about someone who can offer you the full range of treatment options. A good place to start is the National Association for Continence (NAFC) at 1-800-BLADDER. This organization keeps a current directory of people who are active in continence care. You may also call the Society of Urologic Nurses and Associates (SUNA) at 609-256-2335. They have a division of nurses who address continence problems. The American Urologic Association (AUA) at 410-727-1100 also keeps a roster of urologists active in incontinence care as does the American College of Obstetricians and Gynecologists (ACOG) at 202-638-5577. Two other large professional groups that have members who may provide treatment but not a diagnosis are the Wound, Ostomy, and Continence Nurses Society (enterostomal therapists or ET nurses) and the American Physical Therapy Association. Contacting one of these organizations will help you locate a provider who can give you the type of care you need.

Organizations That Can Help You Find a Continence Provider	
National Association for Continence (NAFC)	1-800-BLADDER
Society of Urologic Nurses and Associates (SUNA)	1-609-256-2335
American Urologic Association (AUA)	1-410-727-1100
American College of Obstetricians and Gynecologists (ACOG)	1-202-638-5577
Wound, Ostomy, and Continence Nurses (WOCN)	1-888-224-WOCN
American Physical Therapy Association (APTA)	1-703-684-APTA

What You Should Find Out

Once you receive some names, feel free to contact the provider's office to ask questions about the care you might expect to receive on your first visit and on subsequent visits. Ask if the provider uses some of the treatments that will be discussed in the later chapters as a matter of routine. Not all offices can offer all treatments, but they should be willing to refer you to someone who can provide the treatment you need. Remember that at this stage you do not necessarily want a good surgeon, but rather a good investigator who is willing to work with you. The probability is that at most only about 40 percent of those seeking care for their incontinence will absolutely need a surgical procedure.

Because insurance coverage for incontinence can vary greatly, make certain you know the terms of your policy before seeking care. Some insurance companies require preauthorization for certain devices or if you choose to see a provider who is not in your network. There is nothing worse than getting a huge bill that has been denied payment because you did not follow the procedures laid out by your plan. All insurance companies have a number that can be called for preauthorization. If you are unsure of your coverage, you can call ahead to make certain the treatment you are thinking about is covered.

As a rule, insurance companies will not give an answer about an individual's coverage to the health care provider's office, but they must tell you, the consumer, what is covered. So although it is tempting to ask the office to inquire for you, you will get the best answer by calling yourself. You may request that the answer be in a written form so that there is no misunderstanding. When calling, expect to talk to at least two or three people at your insurance company before finding the person who can answer your question. Your insurance company may ask you to get additional information from your provider describing what might occur during your visits. The insurance company may ask both your primary provider and your specialist to write letters requesting coverage for your care. The time you spend on the phone collecting this information can be frustrating and very time-consuming. However, it is only a fraction of the time spent by your provider's office obtaining coverage for your care. Time is money, so once you've gone through this process, you will understand why insurance premiums are so high! When seeking this care, you will learn a lot about the insurance game.

Obtaining Coverage When Care Is Denied

Ask the office you are thinking of visiting if they will help you obtain insurance coverage for procedures that may have spotty coverage such as biofeedback or pelvic muscle stimulation. If the office states that helping obtain maximum coverage for these procedures and devices is routine for them, then this is an office with which you want to be associated. When a specific device or procedure is not covered, going to the customer service representative of your insurance plan may be beneficial. If you can show that the alternative is more expensive (for example, surgery), most plans will bend on the issues. Another alternative is to ask permission to try a treatment for six to eight weeks. At that point, a letter must go to your insurance provider stating your progress and whether further visits are needed and for what length of time. Occasionally, an insurance provider will state that the conservative treatments are experimental treatments. In this case, your specialist must provide them with the codes or the approved numerical designations that insurance companies use to enter data into their computers. As long as the device or the procedure has a code and is FDA approved, it has been accepted as routine practice by international agreement.

Insurance companies that follow Medicare guidelines may be the most difficult to work with, since Medicare frequently does not cover care associated with incontinence except for testing and surgical procedures. Although incontinence is most probable in those age 65 and older, Medicare has a good reason not to cover this care because the costs would be astronomical. Although the government wheels move slowly, the conservative treatments are under scrutiny for coverage at this time as the Agency for Health Care Policy and Research (AHCPR) panel unequivocally stated in 1996 that conservative treatments should be used first.

As a last resort, you can always ask your employer to go to bat for you on this issue. Often, just a note from the personnel department is enough to get insurers to change their minds about covering a certain therapy. Insurers are under great pressure to provide the best package of care to their customers: your employer.

Obtaining Referrals for Covered Care

Once you've selected a provider, you need to think about what you need for your insurance company to assure coverage of your care. Check your policy. In a managed care plan, where you have a small office visit copay and have prepaid the bulk of your care, you may need a referral to not only see a specialist, but depending on how tightly your plan is controlled, you may need permission from your primary care provider to obtain care outside of your network. The referral will specify how many times you may be seen and during what time frame. You may need to call the specialist's office you want to visit to get this information for your primary care provider. Generally, the primary provider's office generates the referral and sends it ahead of your appointment to the specialist's office. You might want to check with the office before your first visit to make sure they have received the referral. If they have not received the referral, it is up to you to get it or deliver a copy of the original to the office on your first visit. Going to a provider outside of your network may require your primary provider's help if the insurance denies permission, as your primary provider will need to write the medical director of the plan stating that the care you need is not provided within the plan.

Often, you may go to an "outside" provider for one visit to assess the situation and develop a treatment plan, but then the plan may refuse further visits on the grounds that the care is available within the plan. This obstacle usually can be overcome by creative thinking and arming yourself with the knowledge of the conservative therapies. For example, if you are looking for a biofeedback provider, your plan may tell you that the service is provided through an affiliated psychologist. However, the psychologist is normally working with patients whose problems are much different. In this case, your plan would have little choice but to send you to an outside provider once you've explained the difference.

At times, the plan will have contracts with certain providers who you must see. However, most plans allow for a second opinion. Although you might need to see two specialists to get to the one you want to see in the first place, it is well worth it to obtain payment for your care, as this care is quite expensive if paid for out of pocket.

Checklist to Complete Before Going to Your Provider

- Did I remember to try all the suggestions in Chapter 3?
- Have I completed my diary?
- Do I want surgery right away or would I like to try nonsurgical procedures?
- Did I call one of the organizations listed previously to locate a health care provider of conservative therapies in my area?
- Have I called the provider's office to find out what is available to me?
- Have I checked with my insurance plan to make sure my care will be covered?
- Did I obtain the necessary referrals if my plan is an HMO (health maintenance organization) type of plan?
- Have I called my previous providers to obtain all my medical records such as lab work, diagnostic tests, notes, and X-rays?

Now that you've learned about how to pick a specialist and get coverage for your care, it is time to examine the alternatives available to you.

FIVE

What to Ask Your Health Care Provider

"If you let decisions be made for you,
you will be trampled."
—BETSY WHITE

Who's Who In Incontinence

When choosing a specialist to help deal with your incontinence, there are a number of factors you will need to consider to obtain the most appropriate care for your situation. Generally, there are five sets of providers giving this type of care. It is important to realize that all continence care, assuming that pathology has been eliminated, is elective in nature, which means that you have a choice in the type of care and procedures you undergo.

Urologists and gynecologists are physicians who receive training in the management of pelvic disorders. Both may go through extra training to become further specialized in the treatment of incontinence. Most are well versed in the surgical management of incontinence and many of their practices can provide conservative treatments.

Both of these groups may have nurses working with them who are familiar with the conservative treatments such as biofeedback, pelvic muscle stimulation (a device used to strengthen the pelvic muscles), or devices such as pessaries and catheters that are used in the management and treatment of this problem. Many nurses working in this area have specialized training and certification in the field of urology (CURN) or skin care and continence treatment (C-WOCN). Certification by WOCN and SUNA is voluntary, so keep mind that there is no required curriculum for these nurses, nor do they have to be certified in order to provide this care.

Physical therapists will not be using devices (such as pessaries, which are inserted into the vagina to help support the pelvic organs) for management of incontinence or doing diagnostic testing. It is not within the scope of their practice. However, the muscle work they do is superb, and if properly trained in these techniques, they provide excellent care.

The last group of continence care providers are nurse practitioners. In their training, nurse practitioners are taught about chronic incontinence and have the ability to order diagnostic tests and medications in most states. Nurse practitioners also have voluntary certification in urology. Most nurse practitioners in this field can insert and care for pessaries and devices, as well as treat incontinence using pelvic stimulation. They can do biofeedback, perform much of the testing, and perform a physical exam, so often their care is covered by insurance and in many states they are able to practice without the supervision of a physician. They do not perform surgery and are not able to do some specific tests, such as cystoscopy (looking into the bladder), although they can refer you for these tests. Nurse practitioners, as well as other nurses specially trained in this field, will take a holistic view of your incontinence and evaluate fluid intake and lifestyle factors as well as recommend products and management strategies. Usually, they follow the patients through the evaluation, treatments, and, if necessary, postsurgical care.

What to Expect

Regardless of who is providing your care, there are a number of tests you should expect to receive and certain information you should be prepared to give in order to receive the best possible care. The first visit should include a lengthy discussion of your problem. You should be prepared to provide information on how often you are going to the bathroom during the day and at night, when you are leaking, what things make the leaking better or worse, and what

Providers and Their Abilities						
Provider	*Surgery*	*Work-up*	*Cystoscopy*	*CMG Testing*	*Diagnosis*	*Biofeedback*
Gynecologists	Yes	Yes	Maybe	Yes	Yes	Maybe
Urologists	Yes	Yes	Yes	Yes	Yes	Maybe
Nurse Practitioners	No	Yes	No	Yes	Yes	Yes
Nurses	No	Sometimes	No	If physician is present	No	Maybe
Physical Therapists	No	No	No	No	No	Yes

things seem to make you leak. The provider will question you closely about the urine stream characteristics, whether you've had a history of urinary tract infections or stones, whether you've ever seen blood in your urine, had pain or discomfort when urinating, or if the urine looks cloudy. You will be asked about the foods, fluids, and medications (prescribed, over the counter, and herbal) you consume. You will be asked about your surgical, medical, childbirth, and sexual histories. After all the questions, usually a physical exam will be done at this visit, including a pelvic examination, a rectal exam to help evaluate your muscle tone, and/or a prostate exam if you're a male. A urine specimen will be collected to check for infection, blood, or diabetes.

This visit will be long. You should come prepared with lists of previous medical procedures you have undergone, illnesses, medications, and a diary. Then there will be time for you to ask questions. Depending on what you and the physician or nurse practitioner decide, you may be started on a treatment at that visit or may be asked to return for further testing.

Testing

Urological tests for incontinence are usually done in the office or at the local hospital and typically don't cause a great deal of discomfort or pain, nor are they very lengthy. Sometimes, physicians or nurse practitioners will treat incontinence for a short time if they are fairly certain of incontinence type after taking your history and performing a physical exam. However, if there is a question regarding the type of incontinence, further testing will be done to help determine the proper treatment course. The most common testing is urodynamics. These tests measure the pressures in the bladder while filling it with water through a catheter (or tube) inserted into the urethra and while you are emptying the bladder. The test attempts to mimic what is happening to you at home, so don't be embarrassed when you leak.

Leaking during these tests makes your provider very happy, as it is helpful in making a diagnosis. The tests may be done using X-ray or in an office without X-ray. The X-rays are usually moving pictures rather than a single shot, so they can give information about how your bladder neck opens when you void. Adding X-rays gives a visual picture that corresponds to the pressure testing, but it is not necessary in most cases to get a fairly accurate picture of what is happening to you.

Urodynamic testing is usually done by a specially trained nurse or a technician, but the ordering physician or nurse practitioner is usually available during the actual test and is often able to tell you what was found immediately after the test. There is no special preparation for urodynamic studies. Your physician may request that you not take medications that affect your bladder for several days before the test in order to get a clearer picture of what is happening. You will need to check this out prior to your tests.

No anesthesia is given, so in most cases you can eat before coming to the testing site and leave immediately afterward with no restrictions on your activities. You may also be asked to come with a comfortably full bladder to the test, because the provider may want to do a uroflow prior to the test to see how you void without a catheter inside your bladder. If this is the case, don't go to the bathroom on the way to the test without checking with your provider first. Otherwise, you may need to wait until your bladder refills before the test can begin.

The backbone of urodynamic testing is a cystometrogram or CMG. This test measures the pressure in your bladder while it is filling and while you are emptying it. This information will let your provider know how much urine your bladder holds, how well it senses filling, how stretchable it is, when it leaks, whether it is irritable, and how strongly it contracts when emptying. A tiny catheter (a hollow tube) is inserted into the urethra about 1 inch into the bladder. This might pinch slightly when the tube is inserted, but then is usually very comfortable after the tube is in place. The insertion of the catheter is the most uncomfortable part of the test. The actual insertion takes about 30 seconds, although the technician will need to prepare your bottom in a sterile fashion before inserting the catheter so that no germs are introduced into the bladder. Once the catheter is in place, it is taped to your leg. Usually another tube similar to the first catheter is placed either into the vagina or into the rectum in order to measure how much pressure is placed on your bladder by your belly. This helps the technician decide if the bladder is irritable or if the increased pressure is from laughing or talking.

Finally, sometimes the provider orders an electromyelogram or EMG. This test is used to study the activity of the pelvic floor. It helps determine whether the muscles are contracting and relaxing when they are supposed to, as well as the general activity of these muscles while the bladder is filling. Sticky patches, similar to the patches used to monitor your heart during an electrocardiogram (EKG), are placed on the skin on either side of the anus to collect the information about the activity of the pelvic muscles. These patches will stay in place throughout the testing.

Once all these tubes and patches are in place, the testing will probably take about a half hour. The bladder is slowly filled with sterile fluid through the catheter that is in your bladder. Depending on the temperature and how fast the fluid is run, you may feel the fluid filling your bladder. During this time, you will be either lying down or sitting up. You will be asked to report when you would start thinking about going to the bathroom, when you would actually go to the bathroom, and when you cannot hold it anymore. You may also be asked to cough, bear down, or jump in place in order to provoke leaking. Once the technician is satisfied with the quality of the information obtained, you will be asked to void on a special mechanical toilet with the tubes and patches in place. This will help determine how well your bladder and pelvic muscles work together to empty your bladder.

Another test occasionally used in the evaluation of incontinence is cystoscopy. This test is usually done in the physician's office using a flexible scope to actually look at the walls of the bladder and the urethra. If the physician suspects something other than structural problems or weak muscles, he or she may choose to do this test with you under a general anesthetic. These concerns usually arise from other tests, such as the urinalysis, or from your history. Interstitial cystitis (longstanding irritation of the bladder wall) may be one such condition that warrants cystoscopy with anesthesia. Another instance may be if your doctor suspects cancer in your bladder. With an anesthetic the suspicious area can be removed for further evaluation.

Usually cystoscopy is done in the office with numbing jelly placed into your urethra prior to introducing the scope. Generally, no special preparation is needed if the procedure is done in the office. You can plan on going home right away and resuming your normal activities. You may be given antibiotics to prevent a bladder infection.

Other X-rays may be done if the analysis of the urine shows blood or if the physician suspects you may have stones. However, these tests are not necessary for the routine treatment of incontinence.

Common Tests for Bladder Problems

- Urine Analysis and Culture (UA/UC): looks for infection in urine; also lets physician know about chronic inflammation, crystals, and blood or sugar in the urine
- Uroflow study: evaluates how strong the stream is; used as a screening test for obstruction
- Residual urine: can be done by catheter or bladder scan; checks how much urine is left in bladder after voiding
- Cystometrogram (CMG): measures capacity, irritability, stretchability, and leaking of bladder
- Electromyelogram (EMG): evaluates pelvic muscle function
- Cystoscopy: evaluates the wall of the bladder; provider actually looks at the bladder wall

---

Evaluation of incontinence is often complicated, but it is the cornerstone to good, effective treatment. Let your provider know early in the decision making how far you are willing to go in the treatment of your problem. Open communication is very important during the entire evaluation and treatment process.

SIX

Medication Use

"Change is not made without inconvenience, even from
better to worse."
—SAMUEL JOHNSON

Before Starting Medication

There are numerous medications to treat incontinence. In general,
they are used to treat urge incontinence (UI), a few are used to treat
stress urinary incontinence (SUI), and occasionally they are used to
treat overflow incontinence. Since overflow incontinence is often
caused by blockage of the urethra, most treatments are aimed at re-
lieving this blockage. If you are a man with an enlarged prostate, your
physician may use medication to help shrink the prostate, such as finasteride (Proscar), or medication to help relax the urethra, such as
terazosin (Hytrin), doxazosin (Cardura) or tamsulosin hydrochloride
(Flomax). The main side effect of these medications is lightheaded-
ness when going from a laying or sitting position to standing. Rarely
is impotence (an inability to achieve erection) a side effect.

If it seems that the problem causing the blockage is overactive
pelvic floor muscles, a muscle relaxant may be used such as cycloben-
zaprine (Flexeril) or lorazepam (Ativan) and occasionally diazepam
(Valium). The main side effect of these medications is drowsiness. If
diabetes, multiple sclerosis, or some other neurologic disease is the
cause of overflow incontinence, self-catheterization may be prescribed
(this technique is described elsewhere in the book).

Patients with functional incontinence have difficulty getting to the bathroom because of physical limitations. Medication to decrease pain or the stiffness in arthritic joints may indirectly improve continence by allowing you to move better. More often, the treatment in these cases is to bring the toilet, commode, or urinal closer to the patient.

The bladder wall and urethra have special receptors for some chemicals that are found in the bloodstream. These chemicals will either cause the bladder and urethra to contract or relax. We can take advantage of this by counteracting what is happening. For example, if your bladder is overactive, you may be given a medication to activate the receptors that cause the bladder to relax. If you are given a trial of treatment for your bladder problem with medication, plan on keeping your provider updated on your progress or lack of progress. You may need to try several different medications before you find one that works for you.

With any medication, interactions and side effects are possible. Therefore, it is imperative that your health care provider know all medications that you are taking, even the ones that you get without a prescription. It is also very important that you know the potential benefit for your type of incontinence so that you can decide if the potential risks are worth it to you. Remember that you always have a choice. Prior to starting medication for your bladder problems, it is important that you are evaluated to determine the type of incontinence that you have, because taking these medications can make some types of incontinence worse.

Urge Incontinence Medication

Medications used to treat urge incontinence (UI) basically help your bladder to "relax" so that it can hold more urine, letting you make fewer trips to the bathroom. The primary side effects are dry mouth, constipation, blurred vision, and fatigue. You may experience none or all of these side effects and they may or may not be bothersome. Constipation, while it may not seem to be the most bothersome to you, can actually worsen urge incontinence, so it may be necessary to stop the medication or use a stool softener. These medications should not be used or should be used with caution in people with narrow-angle glaucoma, ulcerative colitis, urinary obstruction, myasthenia gravis, or severe heart disease. In general, a two- to four-week trial of medication is warranted to assess effectiveness unless, of course, the side effects are intolerable. Often, if one drug is not tolerated or is ineffective, another will be tried. If you're tired of drugs or if they are not working, let your provider know. Only you can say if the treatment is effective enough for you.

Medications For Stress Incontinence

Occasionally, medications are tried for stress incontinence. They are effective approximately 10 to 20 percent of the time, and like medications for urge incontinence, they work only for as long as you take them. The primary side effects are increased heart rate, feelings of agitation, or worsening of high blood pressure. If you have any of these conditions, you should only take these medications under close supervision from your health care provider.

Specifics about Medications

Let's talk more specifically about the different medications:

- Oxybutynin (Ditropan)—for UI: an antispasmodic that decreases the ability of the bladder to squeeze and delays the onset of the first bladder contraction; 10 to 50 percent cure or reduction in symptoms according to a study performed by the Agency for Health Care Policy and Research (AHCPR) in 1992.
- Oxybutynin XL (Ditropan XL)—for UI: a new formulation of oxybutynin, taken once daily instead of three times per day; incidence of side effects less than with standard oxybutynin.
- Tolteradine (Detrol)—for UI: works similarly to oxybutynin, but with fewer reported side effects.
- Hyoscamine (Levsinex, Levbid)—for UI: similar to oxybutynin except it is the only medication of this type that can be taken on an as-needed basis.

- Dicyclomine (Bentyl)—for UI: similar to oxybutynin, but more traditionally used for intestinal spasms.
- Imipramine (Tofranil)—for UI and SUI: traditionally used as an antidepressant, but has been used in urology for quite some time because the side effects are beneficial to our patients; it decreases the strength of bladder contractions similar to oxybutynin and increases the tone of some of the muscles leading from the bladder.
- Propantheline (Probanthine)—for UI: similar to oxybutynin but response rates are lower at 0 to 50 percent cure or reduction in symptoms.
- Flavoxate (Urispas)—for UI: similar to oxybutynin.
- Phenylpropanolamine—for SUI: found in many decongestants and appetite suppressants, helps to increase the tone of the sphincter muscle that closes the urethra; should be used with caution in men with obstructive symptoms (decreased force of stream, hesitancy) as it can lead to the inability to empty the bladder.
- Pseudoephedrine (Sudafed)—for SUI: similar to phenylpropanolamine, found in many decongestants.
- Terazosin (Hytrin)—for overflow incontinence caused by prostate or urethral blockage: originally marketed for the treatment of high blood pressure; recently also found to have the effect of relaxing the prostate and urethral smooth muscle.
- Doxazosin (Cardura)—same use as terazosin: works similarly to terazosin; both medications may require slowly increasing the dosage to get the desired effect; improvement is usually noted one to two weeks after reaching the maximum dose.
- Tamsulosin (Flomax)—same use as terazosin: works similarly to terazosin and doxazosin, but is first drug of this type specifically for this problem; less need to increase the dose, improvement in symptoms noted as quickly as two to three days after initiation of therapy.
- Finasteride (Proscar)—for treatment of bladder symptoms caused by enlarged prostate: this is the only medication that will decrease the size of the prostate; takes three to six months for maximum effect; few side effects, very low inci-

dence of erection problems; because of the length of time it takes for this medication to work, often it is combined initially with one of the previous three.

- Urecholine—for overflow incontinence due to poor bladder muscle function: this medication helps to increase the strength of the squeeze of the bladder muscle; in our experience it is not very successful.

Is Estrogen For Me?

Many of the incontinence symptoms worsen during menopause. We know that the urethra is embedded in the upper wall of the vagina and develops from the same tissue as the vagina. It also has hundreds of estrogen receptors. Therefore, we can assume that whatever shape the vaginal tissue is in probably holds true for the urethral tissue as well. Although we are unsure of exactly how estrogen works, it is hypothesized to work in several ways. Estrogen is thought to make the tissues surrounding the urethra plumper and more elastic so that the urethra closes more tightly. Softer tissues with good lubrication seem to decrease the sense of irritation and urgency that women may feel as they progress through menopause. Estrogen is also believed to change the pH of the lining of the vagina, making it less likely for bacteria to be able to cause an infection. Finally, it is believed that estrogen helps promote lubrication of the urethra. The lubricant is mucus and helps make the urethra lining sticky; this makes the urethra more effective in the prevention of incontinence.

Although your body continues to produce estrogen throughout your life, estrogen levels begin to decrease in your mid-30s to 40s during perimenopause. During perimenopause, many women notice that the character of their periods change, with bleeding becoming heavier and more clotting occurring. You may also notice that your cycle has become more unpredictable. Your vagina may be drier, you may be more prone to vaginal and urinary tract infections, and intercourse may be uncomfortable unless a lubricant is used. Estrogen levels decrease even more dramatically once you stop menstruating. Shortly afterward, bone density loss accelerates, as does the rate of heart disease.

These changes in disease rates have led scientists to study the effect of estrogen replacement for women, and estrogen replacement has received a lot of press lately. Conflicting studies are released almost annually regarding the benefits of estrogen replacement on the heart and bones and the possible increased risks of uterine and breast cancer. At the present time, we don't know enough about a dose to obtain benefits without the risks. Scientists believe that the risk of heart disease is lower in women who take estrogen. We know that estrogen does offer protection from osteoporosis, but that the dosing needs to be fairly high. Dosing at that level may cause spotting and breakthrough bleeding in women who have stopped cycling. There is evidence that estrogen is related to an increased risk of uterine cancer in those who still have a uterus. The jury is still out on whether estrogen is related to an increased risk of breast cancer and whether that statistic is meaningful, given the much higher rates of heart disease and osteoporosis in older women. It is important to remember that all medications have risks. It is necessary for you to weigh the risks versus the potential benefits of any medication you take.

Although there is no current consensus in the literature that estrogen replacement is beneficial in treating urinary incontinence, most urologists and gynecologists feel that it is beneficial. Usually, if estrogen is being used to treat only urinary symptoms, a very low dose is needed and it is used topically (placed directly into the vagina) either in a cream used two to three times per week or a device shaped like a ring that releases estrogen slowly over three months. There is little to no systemic absorption (no effect on the rest of your body), so usually there are few side effects. If side effects develop, they range from breast tenderness to vaginal irritation and can usually be stopped by decreasing the dose. When used for the treatment of incontinence, it is not unusual to see oral (taken by mouth) and vaginal estrogen used at the same time.

Herbal Remedies

Some people try to use herbal medicines as part of their incontinence treatment. Although some of the herbal medications look promising, keep in mind that the United States does not regulate the production of herbal medication in the same fashion that prescribed drugs are regulated. Therefore, there are very few controlled studies determining the safe dosing, side effects, or purported use for these medications. In addition, the manufacture of these compounds is not regulated, nor are we always sure of the active ingredient. Therefore, the activity of the compound may vary from manufacturer to manufacturer. The last problem with herbals is that we are not sure of their interaction with other drugs you might be taking. Common herbals used in the treatment of urinary problems are listed in the box below. If you choose to use herbals in the treatment of your problem, be certain that you let both your urinary specialist and your primary provider know that you are taking these compounds and then follow their advice.

Herbal Treatments for Incontinence

Herbal Remedies	*Supposed Action**
Bearberry	bladder infections, urinary antiseptic
Bilberry	diuretic
Calendula	antiinflammatory, antiviral
Chamomile	promote urination, relieve spasm
Cranberry	prevent adhesion of *Escherichia coli* (bacteria) to the bladder wall
Dandelion	diuretic
Echinacea	heal infections
Ephedra	diuretic, tighten sphincter (natural form of pseudoephedrine)
Garlic	antibacterial, antifungal, and antiinflammatory
Goldenseal	antiinflammatory
Gotu kola	improve healing, treat urinary tract infections
Hops	decrease spasm, treat urinary tract infections

continued

Kava kava	decrease spasm, treat urinary tract infections
Saw palmetto	decrease urgency and nocturia associated with benign prostatic hypertrophy (BPH)—may help with overflow incontinence caused by prostate blockage

*The exact effects, doses, and interactions of these herbal supplements are unknown at this time. Before taking them, check with your physician regarding their safety.

As you can see, there are many drugs and herbal remedies, and often combinations of drugs and herbals are used to treat incontinence. This list is by no means exhaustive, but it does cover the major medications and herbals and side effects. Remember to give any medication a fair trial (two to four weeks)—that is, of course, if the side effects are not too bothersome. If medications aren't helpful or you do not like taking them, speak up. Let your provider know so that you can move on to some other form of treatment. If your provider doesn't offer you any other treatment, move on to another provider who is more amenable to working with you in trying to find an acceptable solution to your incontinence.

Medications That Can Affect the Bladder

If you are taking any of the following medications, be sure to ask your pharmacist how they can affect your bladder:

- Medications for your heart, including blood pressure medications
- Medications for anxiety, depression, or insomnia
- Medications to relieve pain or muscle spasm
- Medications to speed up or slow down smooth muscles such as your heart, stomach, or colon
- Hormone therapy medications
- Alcohol, caffeine
- Antiinflammatory medications
- Sinus medications

SEVEN

Conservative Treatment Alternatives

"Nothing is more powerful than a habit."
—Ovid

Not everyone needs or wants a surgical procedure for their incontinence. In fact, most urologists and gynecologists will now suggest conservative options before considering surgery. Many HMO (health maintenance organization) insurance companies also require that the patient has failed other management options before approving surgery. This chapter will cover these options, how they are used, how they are chosen, and what are your chances of success.

Kegel Contractions or Pelvic Muscle Exercises

Conservative therapy options started with Dr. Arnold Kegel in the late 1940s. A gynecologist by trade, Kegel noticed that women who had stronger pelvic muscles recovered from the trauma of childbirth much more quickly than those who didn't. He had his patients do a simple exercise, the Kegel contraction, that used an isotonic contraction to rebuild the pelvic muscle. Curious as to whether this exercise actually strengthened the muscle, he then devised a way to measure the strength of the contraction using a simple manometer (a device that measures pressure)—called a *perinometer*—that was inserted into the vaginal vault to measure the pressure exerted by the pelvic muscle when contracting. This idea of pelvic muscle strength measurement became the basis of biofeedback. Eventually, as more work was done in muscle electrophysiology and with the advent of computer technology in the late 1960s and early 1970s, the electrical signal generated by a muscle at work became the accepted standard of measurement. Patients in research labs were connected to computers to ascertain the strength of the muscle. As further work was done in this field, researchers noticed that patients were able to correct errors in muscle use by watching the computer screen and working to change the pattern of the electrical signal. With this realization, biofeedback was born.

Biofeedback

Biofeedback is loosely interpreted by people in the field, depending on what type of equipment is being used. According to *Merriam Webster*, biofeedback is "a technique that enables an individual to gain voluntary control over involuntary body functions by observing electronic measurements of those functions." If the therapist uses a temperature gauge (a thermistor), an audio signal, an electronic wave form, or a digital readout—as long as the signal is collected electronically—the therapist is doing a form of biofeedback. You are a good candidate for biofeedback if you are able to follow directions, are willing to work faithfully at the assigned exercises on a daily basis at home, and have little to no neurologic damage to the pelvic floor.

Biofeedback sessions usually take place in an office setting. However, many therapists take their equipment on the road and can do sessions in people's homes or in satellite clinics. Biofeedback therapists are usually nurses, physical or occupational therapists; however, there are psychologists and physicians who also use these techniques. Before being seen by a therapist, be certain that you have been thoroughly evaluated as described previously, which means you will need to see either a urologist or a gynecologist before going to the therapist. Some primary physicians prefer that you attempt a short course of therapy (six to eight weeks) before a more complicated work-up is done by a specialist.

Before beginning therapy, check the qualifications of your therapist. He or she should be certified to practice in this field. Nurses will have either CURN, C-WOCN, C-BT, or C-NP after their names. Physical therapists will have PT after their names. Look at the office. Is it quiet, clean, and organized? Do you keep your internal sensor (one-person use only)? If your therapist keeps your internal sensor between appointments, is it cleaned immediately after each use with soap and water before repackaging in an individual box or bag labeled with your name or number? Presently, there are no internal electrodes approved for reuse between patients. If the therapist uses external electrodes, are the wires kept clean or changed between patients? Are the wires cleaned with an approved cleaner? If reusable single-person surface electrodes are used, are they also kept individually packaged for you?

The purpose of biofeedback therapy should be explained to you, baseline readings should be taken and interpreted for you, and a copy should be made available for insurance coverage. The first session may take as long as one hour, especially if you are new to the therapist. At an initial biofeedback appointment, the therapist may do a physical exam including a pelvic exam. Rather than looking for pathology, the therapist is looking for your muscle strength and tender spots, as well as whether you understand how to do a Kegel contraction. Depending on these findings, the therapist will either choose an internal or an external sensor. An internal sensor is placed inside the vaginal vault like a tampon or, in males, in the rectum. Your therapist may choose to use skin patches to collect the muscle activity instead of the internal sensor. Either system provides adequate information. Patches will be placed on your abdomen to monitor your abdominal muscles while you are working on your contractions to ensure you are not using the wrong muscles. These sensors are designed to be comfortable, so tell your therapist if they are not. Remember that these sensors just collect the electrical activity of the pelvic muscles. They do not cause your pelvic muscles to contract on their own. Once you are connected to the machine, the therapist will have you lie quietly while he or she collects a resting baseline reading and then will ask you to do a number of maneuvers such as coughing, pulling in your belly, doing "quick flicks" (contracting your muscles strongly for a short time) and 10-second Kegel contractions. The therapist will then review your work, make suggestions for improvement, and will see if the improvement helps increase your strength.

The therapist will collect much of the same information you related to your physician or NP, so it helps to keep copies of this information to bring to the first appointment. Most therapists will do between one and five sessions to observe progress. The possibility of more sessions should be scrutinized as to whether this is the right treatment for you. Follow-up sessions usually last 30 to 45 minutes and will include an evaluation of the muscle strength since the last time you were seen and correction of any errors you might be making. With each session, the number of repetitions of exercises should increase as well as the hold time. Additionally, you should be able to start doing these exercises in sitting and standing positions (functional positions) midway through therapy. If your progress is not notable, then biofeedback is probably not a good choice for you.

Expect to be doing the exercises at these numbers and hold times for 12 to 16 weeks. You will be seen every week to two weeks initially, and appointments are gradually decreased to every month or every six weeks as soon as the therapist is certain you know what you are doing. Some therapists encourage clients to use a portable biofeedback device at home. Keep in mind that these devices are usually not covered by insurance. There is some research that shows patients using home trainers get to their goals a little faster; however, it has not been shown that ultimately people using a home trainer are stronger or better at doing their exercises than those who do not use this equipment.

With biofeedback for appropriate candidates, the improvement rates are in the 54- to 87-percent range. You must continue to do these exercises for the rest of your life. Biofeedback is also a useful tool to help you learn how to relax your pelvic muscles in chronic pain syndromes and urgency/frequency syndromes. This biofeedback requires a highly experienced therapist and it is worth going out of your way to find one.

Checklist for Considering Biofeedback Therapy

- Do I want to do exercises every day?
- Am I willing to wait patiently for results for up to three months?
- Has my provider thoroughly explained how the pelvic muscles work and how I can prevent leaking?
- Have I been told how many return visits I will make and how long it will take before I can expect some changes?
- Does my provider have contingency plans if biofeedback doesn't work for me?
- Will I be learning how to do these exercises in any location, position, and at any time?
- Can my provider show me how I've made progress each week?
- Will my provider write my primary physician regarding my treatment and again at the end of treatment?
- Is my provider and the treatment outlined covered by my insurance?

Pelvic Muscle Stimulation

What happens if biofeedback is not helping? Most biofeedback therapists have another useful tool in their arsenal called pelvic muscle stimulation. An electronic device sends a signal to your muscle to contract (Figure 7.1). Rather than just collecting the signals that your muscle puts out, as in biofeedback, the signal to contract is generated by the device and the muscle contracts in response to this signal. Like all electrical devices, the therapist must be trained and experienced in the various applications. This device works well if you do not have the time to invest in biofeedback, if you have neurologic changes to your bladder, or if you have trouble learning how to correctly use your pelvic muscle. Most pelvic muscle stimulation devices can be used to inhibit urgency and urge incontinence with great success, becoming an alternative to medication. With stress incontinence, success rates may approach 85 percent; with urge incontinence, the rate is closer to 50 percent.

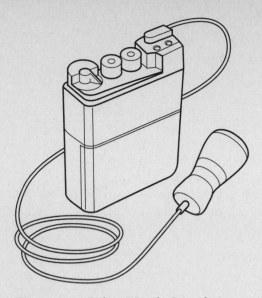

Figure 7.1. Pelvic Muscle Stimulation
System

If you choose pelvic muscle stimulation, you should expect to have an initial work-up by your physician or NP as in biofeedback. Unlike the patient doing biofeedback, the electrode is inserted into the vagina or rectum, so the tissue must be examined for lesions. Vaginal tissue must be soft and stretchy before considering this therapy. While vaginal estrogen helps improve the tissue, there are other lubricants, such as Replens, that can help improve the tissue in women who can't use estrogen or would prefer not to use it. There is no skin preparation for patients using a rectal electrode. If a patient has recently had either vaginal or rectal surgery, the surgical site must be completely healed prior to using an internal electrode. Mothers who recently delivered vaginally must obtain the okay from their gynecologist before starting this therapy. Patients with neurologic diseases such as MS must be followed very closely when using this therapy as their sensation is not good and the condition of their skin must be monitored regularly. Finally, patients who have a pacemaker must not use this therapy because the pelvic stimulation might override their pacemaker.

Usually during the first visit, the therapist will review your case with you. If the therapist has equipment on the premises, fitting of the electronic device will occur on the first visit as well. However, most of the time, these devices are ordered after the first visit because approval from the insurance company must be obtained.

At a visit, once the electrode is inserted, the therapist will slowly raise the settings on the channel until the appropriate sensation is felt. This is a little scary for most people, because the device is actually sending an electrical current to the muscle to contract the muscle directly. Gradually, the setting will be adjusted until you have a comfortable yet strong contraction. This direct contraction of the muscle is why this type of device works so well for patients who cannot initiate a pelvic muscle contraction. With this therapy, the device does the work for you. When using it, there should not be any burning or tingling sensation; if there is, it is generally a sign that the setting is too high or the electrode is not in the correct position. Usually, the first visit lasts about 45 minutes to an hour in order to teach you about the device. Later visits are much shorter and generally just involve checking your progress and readjusting the settings.

After the initial visit, the therapist may see you in 1 or 2 weeks to determine if you are using the device correctly and if any adjustments in the settings need to be made. The therapist might only see you for one or two more visits, spaced 4 to 6 weeks apart. At home you will be using the machine either daily or every other day. The machine is typically used every day, but an alternative protocol is to use it for two 15-minute treatments every other day. Both protocols are effective. Like biofeedback, expect to use the device regularly for 12 to 16 weeks. At the end of treatment, some patients continue to use the device; others use it intermittently, doing Kegel contractions instead to maintain their continence.

Neocontrol

The Neocontrol pelvic floor therapy system is a new treatment for stress urinary incontinence. It was approved for use by the Food and Drug Administration (FDA) in June 1998. This system uses magnetic stimulation of nerves to strengthen the pelvic muscles. The magnet is in the seat of a special chair and is able to penetrate clothing. The magnet causes the nerves to your pelvic muscles to become "excited," which causes the muscles to contract (squeeze).

Therapy involves two 20-minute sessions per week for 8 weeks. There is no probe to place into your vagina or rectum, and because the magnet is able to penetrate clothing, you do not need to undress. The success rate of this therapy is 75 percent, that is, these women were completely dry or significantly improved. Ninety percent of women undergoing this treatment would recommend it to a friend. Neocontrol is for people with mild to moderate stress incontinence. It does not teach you how to contract your muscle voluntarily as biofeedback and pelvic stimulation do. It does help to improve the bulk and strength of these muscles. We do not have long-term results as this therapy is so new.

At this point, as providers are unsure of insurance coverage, most candidates are paying out of pocket and are reimbursed if the insurance company covers the therapy. This is not unusual for new treatments. The cost of the 16 sessions ranges from $700 to $1500 depending on where you live. Studies are currently being done to evaluate the effectiveness of Neocontrol for urge incontinence, sexual dysfunction, and postprostatectomy incontinence.

Considering Pelvic Muscle Therapy?

Answer these questions:

- Am I comfortable touching my vagina or rectum?
- For women, have I ever used a tampon or suppositories in the past?
- Can I find 15 minutes twice a day to faithfully do my treatment?
- Am I willing to devote 12 to 16 weeks to therapy?
- Did my health care provider explain how I can use what I learn in treatment and apply it to everyday life?
- Does my provider have contingency plans should this treatment not work for me?

continued

- Do I have a pacemaker?
- Is my vagina or rectum particularly sore or tender?
- If nerve damage is causing my incontinence, am I comfortable using this type of device for the rest of my life?
- Have I been told how many visits I will need, how long therapy will take, and how my progress will be assessed?
- Am I willing to pay for the device if it is not covered by my insurance ($400 to $1500)?

Vaginal Weights or Cones

Another useful device that takes advantage of the Kegel contraction is a set of pelvic muscle weights or cones. These tampon-like devices can be inserted into the vagina and the pelvic muscle is contracted to hold them in place. They are usually worn for 15 minutes once or twice a day. The idea is that when you feel the cone begin to slip out of place, you will contract the pelvic muscle to prevent it from slipping out of the vagina. These cones are a nice adjunct to therapy, but cone use assumes that you can already contract the pelvic muscle correctly. Depending on how weak the pelvic muscle is, you may be told to start with the lightest cone and only sit for 5 minutes with it in place, gradually increasing to 15 minutes over several days. As you begin to keep the cone in place during functional activities such as showering and walking, you will be asked to increase the cone weight until you can again hold it in place for 15 minutes. At the end of treatment, you can choose to continue to use the cones daily or just do Kegel contractions. Success rates vary, depending on who you ask. Cone use requires only an initial evaluation and a follow-up visit. The therapist must be certain that vaginal tone is equal on both sides so that you cannot cheat by having the cone fall into a pocket created by the weaker vaginal wall.

Other Options

The above treatments actually change the way the pelvic muscle functions and, with the exception of vaginal weights, can be used by both men and women. If you have no improvement using exercise, there are some other devices that can be used to improve the anatomic position of a woman's organs so that leaking is less likely to occur. There are three devices that fall into this category: bladder neck prostheses, continence rings, and pessaries.

Pessaries

A pessary is a device inserted into the vagina to support the pelvic organs in the proper position. There is evidence that pessary-like devices, to hold the uterus in place after prolapse, were used during the Classical Greek and Roman times. Both Hypocrites and Celsus describe the use of these devices in their writings. Pomegranates, potatoes, string balls, and sponges have been used at various times throughout history as pessaries. Our grandmothers may have used many of these devices before surgical procedures became popular. Like a diaphragm, a pessary is inserted deeply into the vaginal vault. Once in place, it takes up excess tissue and supports the organs above it in a more anatomically correct position. When placing anything in the vagina, the vaginal tissues must be in good shape, and because these devices stay in place, the patient must have good sensation to the vaginal vault.

Pessaries come in all shapes and sizes and can be used by anyone whose incontinence is related to poor support. Pessaries are prescribed and must be fitted initially by a nurse practitioner, physician, or nurse under the supervision of a physician. They are used as an alternative to surgery, as a temporary fix while a patient awaits surgery, or as a diagnostic tool to see if a planned procedure really does solve the incontinence problem.

Continence Rings

Continence rings, refined in the last few years, use a bump of extra material at the base of the bladder to help press the bladder neck closed. They are inserted in a slightly different fashion than a pessary and actually support the bladder neck rather than organs above the ring. The cost ($30 to $60), care, and prescribing of continence rings are similar to pessaries. The difference between a continence ring and a pessary is in the intended use. A continence ring is specifically designed to occlude the urethra and support the bladder neck, while a pessary provides more generalized support. The fitting and the office visit are similar to a pessary fitting.

Bladder Neck Prostheses

A bladder neck prosthesis functions much like a continence ring; however, the bladder neck prosthesis holds up the tissue on either side of the urethra rather than occluding the bladder neck. A bladder neck prosthesis must be removed daily for cleaning. These devices must be fitted by a provider who receives training from the manufacturer of the device. Bladder neck prostheses are quite a bit more expensive than pessaries and must be preapproved by your insurance company.

General Information About Vaginally Placed Devices

These devices, although tricky to fit properly, work immediately in improving incontinence if the fit is appropriate. Appointments to fit a pessary, continence ring, or bladder neck prosthesis are very similar. Initially the physician or nurse practitioner will assess the vaginal vault using a speculum, looking inside the vault to determine the condition of the skin. Small cuts and infection must be investigated. If the tissue is a healthy pink and is intact, the fitting can proceed. If the tissue looks atrophic, you will be sent home with a prescription for vaginal estrogen for three to four weeks. The estrogen will help plump up the tissue so that wearing the pessary is not uncomfortable. If you choose not to use estrogen, or if estrogen is contraindicated because of a history of breast cancer, you must use an alternate non-estrogen-based cream or a lubricant to enhance the vaginal mucosa and maintain its pH. Your health care provider can help you choose a suitable cream.

The day the device is fitted, there is no special preparation. Generally, it is fitted with a moderately filled bladder as the provider wants to see if you leak after it is in place. When fitting the device, you will be in a legs-up position just like you are for a vaginal exam. Some providers smear the vaginal vault with numbing jelly so that inserting and removing the device is more comfortable. It often takes two or three tries before a suitable device is found. Once the provider is satisfied with the fit, you will be asked to walk around, squat, and cough to make sure it stays in place and fits comfortably. If it is the appropriate treatment and the right size, leaking should not occur or should be significantly less than what it had been previously. Most providers will have you attempt to learn how to take the device out before leaving their office and many will ask you to return to the clinic in a few days to make sure all is well. These devices should be barely felt or not felt at all if they fit properly. You should not have problems emptying your bladder nor should you have back or tail-bone pain. If either situation occurs, call your provider immediately.

Depending on the material, either you are trained to remove the device daily for cleaning and reinsertion or you come into the clinician's office every six to eight weeks to have the device removed, cleaned, and the vaginal vault inspected. Depending on the device, you may be able to have intercourse with it in place. If you are still menstruating, the device will have to be removed at the end of your period to be cleaned and reinserted. With the initial fitting, you will be kept in the office until you are able to urinate. If you are unable to tell the device is in place and you are continent, you can be sure it is in correctly. If your device requires daily removal, you may be shown how to remove it at the initial visit. You may be asked to come back in 24 hours so that the vagina can be inspected for irritation. If all is well, you do not need to be seen again until a routine follow-up appointment.

Although the initial fitting is time-consuming, these devices allow patients to avoid surgery for an indefinite period and work well for patients who may not be candidates for other therapies. If you leak only with vigorous activities, you may need to use a device solely during these times. People who might not be aware enough to do an exercise program (Alzheimer's patients, demented patients) may do very well with these devices.

Considering a Pessary?
Answer these questions:

- Am I comfortable having something in my vagina all the time?
- Do I understand how to take care of the pessary?
- Do I realize that I will have an increased risk of vaginal and bladder infections when using a pessary?
- Do I understand that a pessary does not correct a prolapsed uterus or bladder? It only manages the problem.
- Do I understand that if I have back pain or trouble urinating a pessary may not be an option for me?
- Do I realize that fitting a pessary is an imprecise process that may require me to return to the clinic for a corrected fit?
- Do I realize that I will need to return to the clinic regularly (every six to eight weeks) for vaginal exams and for cleaning of the pessary?
- Do I understand how to remove the pessary?
- Can my pessary be used during intercourse?

Containment Options

Containment devices also manage incontinence rather than change the conditions that cause it. These devices include urethral plugs, patches, caps, and catheters. When in place, they decrease the amount of leaking, but the leaking will be as bad as ever when the devices are not in place.

Urethral Plugs

A urethral plug is placed into the urethra and partially into the bladder. When the balloon in the bladder is blown up, the balloon blocks the opening to the bladder and no urine escapes. When the balloon is deflated, the plug is removed and disposed of so that you are able to urinate normally. These devices can be used only under the direction of a gynecologist, urologist, or nurse practitioner. Because the plug actually goes into the bladder, there is a risk of infection and irritation of the urethral wall. It may take some time to become comfortable with placement. In general, most women are able to learn how this is done. The cost (about $1 per use) of this device is fairly high and reserved for people with good cognition, compliance, and dexterity.

External Urethral Occlusion Devices

Urethral caps and patches are very new devices that are applied to the external opening of the urethra to prevent urine leakage. Some are reusable. They are removed each time you urinate and then reapplied before resuming activities. Infection rates are low, but like the plug, it takes time to learn how to use the device correctly. You must have normal mental and hand function. These devices are made for mild to moderate cases of stress incontinence. They are not advisable if you have an irritable bladder, are poorly estrogenized, or are sensitive to feeling the device in place.

Catheters

Catheters are used in some cases of overflow incontinence or very severe urge incontinence. A catheter is a hollow tube inserted into your bladder to drain urine from the bladder. Two types of catheters are used: an indwelling catheter, which remains in place, permanently draining urine around the clock; and an intermittent self-catheterization (ISC) program—that is, you insert a catheter when urine needs to be drained from your bladder and then it is immediately removed. A person needing a catheter should always be under the care of a urologist because the risk of infection and danger of kidney damage can be much higher than normal. Choosing a catheter type and treatment via a catheter is always a complex and a very individual decision. If you have good balance and good hand and mental function, you are a candidate for intermittent self-catheterization. The switch to an indwelling catheter is made if ISC is difficult, so frequent that it is impractical, or poor hand function or balance problems make ISC impossible.

General Information

Office visits are similar for all these devices. Urodynamic testing is usually done, except in the case of external devices, to determine if you are a candidate for a containment device. Generally, there is a lot of teaching involved and you will be asked to return to demonstrate the correct way to insert or place the device and to care for it. With the urethral plug, a fitting may be required. You will also be asked to return to the clinic within a few weeks to determine that you are using the device correctly. Finally, you will be monitored closely for urinary tract infection.

Considering a Containment Device

Answer these questions:

- Do I understand how to use the device and how to clean and care for it?
- Do I understand the purpose of the device?
- Will I need to be on a daily low dose of antibiotics to prevent infection?
- Do I know what to do if I show signs of a urinary tract infection or if I see blood in my urine?
- Do I know the signs and symptoms of a urinary tract infection?
- Do I realize that my bladder and kidney function need to be checked regularly?
- Do I realize that once I start inserting a device into my bladder that my urine is likely to always have bacteria?

EIGHT

Surgical Options

"There are only hints and guesses,
Hints followed by guesses, and the rest
Is prayer, observance, discipline, thought and action."
—T. S. Eliot

Surgical Candidates

There are several surgeries for stress incontinence. The intent is usually
to correct an anatomic defect such as urethral hypermobility or bladder
or uterine prolapse. The assumption is that once the defect is corrected,
the incontinence will be corrected. However, this is not always the case.
A multifaceted problem will require a multifaceted approach. Unless
there is a great degree of prolapse, more conservative measures, such as
biofeedback and pelvic stimulation (Chapter Seven), may be offered as
first-line therapy. Many of you may not choose to be treated conserva-
tively, but these treatment options should at least be offered. Many of
my patients choose to go forward with surgery instead of initial conservative management because they do not feel they will be compliant with
the exercise program. Be honest with yourself. If you don't feel that you
can make that commitment, perhaps surgery is for you. However, there
are several things you should know about these surgical procedures.

Classifications of Surgery

There are three major surgical classifications for stress incontinence:
bulking procedures, bladder-neck suspensions, and slings. The suc-

cess of each of these depends on proper evaluation and patient selection. These procedures have the possibility of failure over time. Next, I discuss the success and failure rates with individual procedure descriptions.

Complications of Surgery

As with any surgical procedure, there is a risk for complications. Death during or secondary to an incontinence procedure is extremely rare, approximately 1 percent. Requiring a blood transfusion is also uncommon—a risk of less than 5 percent. More common complications include the possible development of urge incontinence when it did not exist before. The exact incidence is unknown, but I tell my patients to expect frequency and urgency after surgery that may last up to three months; if it has not subsided by this time, nonsurgical treatments may be undertaken.

Urinary retention or incomplete bladder emptying are also possible complications of surgery. These problems usually last one to two weeks, but can last up to three months. Occasionally, swelling at the surgical site occludes the urethra, or the pelvic muscles become spastic due to the surgical trauma and do not relax appropriately. Urine must be drained through a catheter until this subsides. The bladder is managed by either an indwelling catheter (a hollow tube inserted into the bladder through the urethra and connected to a urine collection bag), a suprapubic tube (a hollow tube placed into the bladder through the abdomen at the time of surgery), or intermittent self-catheterization. Infection is always a risk with any surgery, but with incontinence surgery it tends to be relatively minor, usually a bladder infection that is treated easily with antibiotics. Often, antibiotics are given in an effort to prevent infections.

The Surgeries

As previously stated there are a number of ways to perform surgery for incontinence. The type of surgery you have will depend on what is found during your evaluation, as well as the types of surgery your physician is familiar with and comfortable performing.

Bulking Procedures

Urethral bulking procedures are generally performed in women and men whose internal urethral sphincter is not functioning properly. The women tend to have very little prolapse with a large degree of incontinence. They may also have had previous incontinence surgery or nerve damage to the sphincter from trauma, such as childbirth, hysterectomy, or other pelvic surgery. The men almost always have had some type of pelvic or prostate surgery.

The current most popular bulking agent is a glutaraldehyde cross-linked bovine collagen (Contigen). In women, the procedure is usually done on an outpatient basis without general anesthetic (frequently, only local numbing medications are used). In men, because of their different anatomy, general anesthetic is almost always used. Restrictions after the procedure are minimal. Your doctor may restrict sexual activity for some time after the procedure. Before the Contigen can be injected, a skin test must be performed to make sure that you do not have an allergic reaction. This is done by injecting a small amount of the material under the skin on your arm, which must be observed for one month before proceeding with the urethral injection.

For women, this procedure is done either in the office or in the outpatient surgery department of the hospital. Your legs will be placed in stirrups as they are for your pelvic exam. Your bottom will be washed by the nurse in the room and possibly an anesthetic jelly will be placed into your urethra. After a few minutes, the doctor will place a cystoscope (a lighted telescope) into your bladder. Some use a video camera and will allow you to watch as the procedure is done (you can always close your eyes if you don't want to see). If an anesthesiologist has not given you medication into an intravenous (IV) line, your doctor will inject more numbing medication (usually lidocaine) into your urethra. This is likely to be the most painful part of the procedure and has been characterized by patients as a burning, pressure sensation. Once this step is done, the procedure should not be painful. Contigen is injected while the surgeon is watching until the urethral opening closes; it may take one to three syringes of medication. Then you will likely be asked to urinate before you are allowed to leave. If you are unable to void, you will be taught to catheterize yourself until you are voiding well. Most patients are usually voiding well by the next day. However, to avoid problems with voiding, most physicians will do this procedure in steps. It is not unusual for 3 to 5 injections to be needed. Keep in mind that Medicare may not pay for more than five injections in a series.

For men, the Contigen injection is almost always done in the hospital and anesthesia is administered. The injection is given by either passing the cystoscope through the urethra to the area to be injected or through a small puncture made through the skin on your belly into your bladder. The scope will be placed and passed through the bladder into the urethra, where the collagen will be injected. The scope will then be removed. The routine after this procedure is generally the same as that for women.

The success rate in women is 80 percent after two injection sessions. Once you are dry, you can expect to stay that way for 12 to 24 months, and then the procedure can be repeated. Usually, at least two injection sessions are done before the procedure is pronounced a failure. If there has been no improvement after two sessions, it is not likely that success will occur, and some other form of treatment should be entertained. The success rate for men is 8 to 30 percent. One thing for both men and women to remember is that other procedures can be tried if this one is not successful. Of course, a careful evaluation should be done prior to any procedure.

Fat is another material that is injected as a bulking agent. It is injected in much the same way as Contigen; the difference is that the fat must be removed from you before it can be injected. The fat is usually taken from your belly (it's liposuction, except you probably won't notice a significant change in the way your belly looks). It is then injected into your urethra like Contigen. The success rate is a little lower, but this may be a good alternative for those who are allergic to collagen.

Bladder-Neck Suspensions

Bladder-neck suspensions are done to support the bladder neck (opening of the bladder to the urethra). This surgery uses strong tissue beside the bladder neck as support. In general, sutures are placed into the strong supporting tissue and are either tied to strong tissue inside your pelvis, just above your pubic bone, or they may be secured to your pubic bone by screws. This procedure can be done through an incision in your belly, using scopes through your belly, or vaginally with a small incision above your pubic bone. The surgery has a variety of names; most techniques are named for the person or persons who developed them. Burch, Stamey, Raz, modified Pereyra, Marshall–Marchetti–Krantz, and Vesica are names of the most popular bladder-neck suspensions.

The Burch is done either as an "open" procedure with an abdominal incision or laparoscopically (with a telescope and a camera) through several small abdominal incisions. If the open procedure is done, sutures (strong stitches) are placed in the strong tissue next to the bladder neck and secured to strong tissue at the side of your pelvis, called Cooper's ligament. If done with the scope, either sutures or mesh (artificial tissue) is used. The mesh is attached using clips. According to the *Female Stress Urinary Incontinence Clinical Guidelines Panel Summary Report on Surgical Treatment of Female Stress Urinary Incontinence*, the cure rate of this surgery in the short and long term is fairly good, ranging from 77 to 89 percent and remaining at this level over a five-year period. The open procedure has a much longer track record, but the laparoscopic approach appears to have a comparable success rate. The laparoscopic approach is favorable to many patients because of the shorter recovery time due to less pain from the incision.

Marshall–Marchetti–Krantz (MMK) requires an incision. Sutures are placed in the strong tissue beside the urethra and bladder neck and are then secured to the pubic bone. The success data for this procedure are similar to the Burch according to the same report. The Raz, modified Pereyra, Vesica, and Stamey procedures are all done primarily through the vagina with a small incision made just above the pubic bone. The Stamey uses a small piece of artificial tissue over a suture to help support the bladder neck. The suture is then transferred to the incision over your pubic bone using a special needle. It is either tied or secured to your pubic bone with screws. The Raz, modified Pereyra and Vesica techniques attach sutures directly to your tissue, securing them above or to your pubic bone as in the Stamey procedure. According to the *Clinical Guidelines*, success ranges from 71 to 86 percent initially to 53 to 79 percent at five years.

Sling Procedures

The sling procedure is done primarily through the vagina. A strip of tissue or artificial tissue is used to support the urethra and bladder neck much as a hammock supports you as you recline. The sling acts as a backboard for your urethra during stress maneuvers such as coughing, running, and jumping. It also closes the urethra during these maneuvers.

The material used to "sling" the urethra can be fascia (strong tissue that envelops muscles) or artificial tissue. The fascia can be removed from you or it can be from a tissue bank. The advantage of using banked tissue is that you have a much smaller incision (making your recovery time potentially shorter), the tissue is reliably strong and the surgical time is shortened by 20 to 30 minutes. The disadvantage is that this tissue has been removed from a cadaver (a dead person who is a donor) and there is a slight risk of contracting an infectious disease, although to date no incidents have been reported in the United States. The success rate of the sling, according to the *Clinical Guidelines* ranges from 73 to 89 percent initially to 75 to 89 percent at five to ten years.

After Surgery

The success of these surgeries depends on proper evaluation as well as the experience of your surgeon. You also have some say in the likelihood of success, since you must follow your surgeon's instructions after surgery. You will be hospitalized for up to two days, although possibly not at all. Once you are home, you will probably be more tired than you think you should be. Listen to your body and rest when you feel you should. Your doctor will restrict lifting, asking you not to lift anything heavier than 5 to 10 pounds for six to eight weeks after your surgery. This gives your body time to begin developing scar tissue to help the sutures that are providing the initial support. Doing heavy lifting (including vacuuming and maybe even carrying your purse) increases the risk of breaking the sutures.

Urge Incontinence Procedures

Surgery for urge incontinence and urgency is not done as commonly as surgery for stress urinary incontinence, but according to many studies, those of you with this problem are bothered much more than those with stress incontinence. This is likely because you have no idea of when the overwhelming desire to urinate will hit you or where the closest bathroom will be. The treatments for urgency and urge incontinence include medications, as discussed in Chapter Six, or behavioral and pelvic muscle therapies, as discussed in Chapter Seven. These are first-line treatments and should generally be tried before proceeding with surgery.

Augmentation

If your true bladder capacity has decreased significantly, as with some cases of interstitial cystitis, radiation treatments, and diseases such as tuberculosis or multiple sclerosis, a bladder augmentation may be recommended. (Keep in mind that I said *true* bladder capacity, which is usually measured with you under a general anesthetic so that sensory input [your brain] doesn't interfere.) Bladder augmentation increases your bladder capacity by using a segment of your intestine.

It is possible that after this operation you will be unable to urinate because the ability of your bladder to squeeze has been lost. You should expect to perform intermittent self-catheterization permanently after this type of surgery and be pleasantly surprised if this is not the case. Hospitalization is anywhere from 5 to 10 days if there are no complications. You will have a tube in your nose draining your stomach when you awake from surgery, as well as a tube (catheter) draining your bladder through your belly, and possibly a catheter into your bladder through your urethra. The tube draining your stomach will remain until your intestines begin to work (you pass gas), which may take as long as 3 to 4 days. You will not be allowed to eat while this is in place. The catheter through your urethra will stay until you are up and around in the hospital. The one through your belly into your bladder serves two purposes: to drain your bladder and to allow the nurses and you to irrigate (flush fluid through) your new bladder so that mucus produced by the intestinal segment will not plug your catheter. This catheter will remain in place for 3 to 6 weeks while the new bladder heals. Possible complications from this surgery include problems with the intestinal reconnection or with the attachment of the intestinal segment to the bladder. Complications could require further surgery.

Diversions

Sometime the urinary bladder functions so poorly that it is best to bypass it all together. There are a number of ways this can be achieved, and it is usually your surgeon's preference which diversion you will have if you have chosen this route of management. All diversions use a part of your intestine to collect the urine. There are continent and incontinent diversions. If you have an incontinent diversion, your urine will empty into a collection device that is applied to your skin. This device is a special bag that is fit over the stoma (small portion of intestine exposed on the skin surface). This is the easiest diversion to perform and has the least risk for complication. The complications are the same as those for augmentation plus there is the possibility that the ureter (tube that carries urine from the kidney to the bladder or the intestinal segment) will scar and cause blockage of the kidney. This complication could lead to reoperation.

Continent diversions do not require the use of a collection appliance. Instead, the intestinal segment collects urine just as your bladder would. You have to drain this "bladder" with a catheter that goes into a segment of intestine that has been brought to your skin surface. This type of diversion is generally done for people with good hand function, but who are unable to catheterize their urethra. The complications from this type of surgery are the same as those for augmentation, in addition to the possibility that the continence mechanism might fail, which would require reoperation to correct. Your postoperative course would be similar to that of bladder augmentation.

Sacral Nerve Stimulation

Sacral nerve stimulation is a relatively new procedure that uses a small device to generate an electrical impulse to stimulate nerves from your sacrum (the lowest part of your back). The best thing about this procedure is that you get to test it to make sure it will work for you before you have an operation to have it permanently implanted.

A test stimulation is performed by placing the stimulator wires through your skin into the correct spot in your back. The wires are then attached to an external generator that you wear on your waistband. If your symptoms decrease by 50 percent, you are a candidate for the permanent implant. The permanent device is implanted in the operating room. You will have a general anesthetic and most of the surgery will be done with you lying on your stomach. A small incision is made in your lower back and the stimulating wires are placed; then a pocket is made near your side for the generator and the two are connected (wires plugged into the generator). You may remain in the hospital for a day or two. Sometimes the stimulation is begun before you leave or your doctor may prefer to let you heal a little first. The generator is controlled with a magnet. Patients describe the feeling associated with the stimulation as a buzzing sensation that they quickly become used to; when it is turned off, their symptoms quickly return. As with any surgery complications can arise. The main ones specific to this procedure are related to the device. There is a chance that the connections may fail or that the stimulating wires may shift, not giving you the symptom relief you would expect.

Infections are always a risk whenever an artificial device is used, but with antibiotics they are rarely serious. This procedure is proving to be a relief for many people who have suffered with urgency and have had poor success with other modalities.

Remember that you always have a choice as to whether or not you have surgery. If you are uncomfortable with what your doctor is saying, do not hesitate to get a second opinion.

Considering Surgery

Answer these questions:

- Do I understand what surgery will accomplish?
- Do I understand that there is always a risk that the surgery will not solve the problem and may make it worse?
- Have I undergone urodynamic testing?
- Do I understand that if I cannot void after the surgery I will need to wear a catheter or do intermittent catheterization?
- Do I understand the risks of surgery and the rate of infection?
- Do I know how long I will be unable to work, when I can return to regular activities, and when I can resume exercising and lifting?
- Can I afford to take off of work?

NINE

Treatments Available to Men

"It is part of the cure to wish to be cured."
—SENECA

Twelve million people suffer with incontinence, the majority of whom are women, but men can also have this problem. The reasons for incontinence may differ, but the problem is just as frustrating, embarrassing, isolating, and depressing as it is for women.

Women often believe that incontinence is something they have to live with, whereas men usually realize that it is an abnormality and they readily seek treatment. Men, in general, are incontinent as a consequence of treatment of a pelvic condition, such as an enlarged prostate (benign prostatic hypertrophy or BPH), prostate cancer, or even rectal or colon abnormalities. The types of incontinence men can have are the same as those discussed earlier: stress, urge, overflow, or functional.

To review briefly, stress incontinence occurs during activities that cause a rise in abdominal pressure, such as coughing, sneezing, or jumping. Urge incontinence is leakage that occurs once you have the desire to empty your bladder and have difficulty reaching the bathroom on time. Overflow leakage occurs when the bladder reaches capacity and "spills over." Remember the bucket under the faucet that has been neglected. Functional incontinence occurs when you are unable to reach the bathroom in time due to a broken hip or knee replacement or perhaps because of some other physical or mental disability.

Overflow Incontinence and BPH

Overflow incontinence can occur in men with longstanding BPH. These men generally have had problems going to the bathroom for quite some time. They have complained of difficulty starting the urine stream, slow stream, and the feeling that their bladder is not emptying. If this is the cause of your leakage, you may also be going to the bathroom very frequently during the day and the leakage may occur just at night when your brain isn't focused on your bladder.

Your bladder has undergone quite a few changes to get to this "decompensated" state. The muscles of your bladder thickened to overcome the blockage caused by your growing prostate. This thicker bladder wall allows the bladder to push harder. At first, you may not notice any change in your stream. Over time, your bladder begins to lose its elasticity and is unable to squeeze the urine out because the thickened wall has no stretch. This leads to incomplete emptying of your bladder. As more time passes, your bladder decompensates even further and you may be unable to empty your bladder at all or overflow incontinence may occur.

The treatment is relief of the obstruction, either surgically or by placement of a catheter through the penis or belly to drain the bladder. One thing to remember about surgery is that your bladder may not function properly afterward. Once a bladder has become decompensated, it is very difficult for it to recover its former function. If you are unable to urinate after surgery, you will need to have a permanent catheter, perform intermittent self-catheterization, or perhaps have a diversion surgery as described in Chapter Eight.

Frequency, urgency, and urge incontinence can occur due to BPH, although they are considered irritative symptoms. In most men, these symptoms resolve after treatment for the obstruction. Still, the symptoms do occasionally continue and often treatments such as biofeedback or pelvic muscle stimulation can be instituted (see Chapter Seven).

Prostatectomy for benign prostatic hypertrophy was the mainstay for treatment of blockage of the urethra caused by an enlarging gland until the late 1980s. At that time, many new medications were introduced that are very effective in managing this problem. They are discussed in Chapter Six as medications that may be used to treat overflow incontinence.

Surgery, specifically transurethral resection of the prostate, is the option for men who do not respond to these medications or who have a large prostate. This procedure uses scopes and electric current to remove the portion of the prostate that is blocking the urethra. The surgeon must be very careful not to injure the external sphincter that is very close to the end of the prostate. If the sphincter is injured, incontinence can occur.

Prior to surgery, the prostate had been used to help with urinary control as had the muscles of the urethra known as the internal sphincter. By necessity, the TURP damages the internal sphincter, making it nonfunctional. Many men will have some urgency and frequency immediately after the surgery, but this generally resolves within two to three months, if not sooner. Remember that some of the symptoms of prostate enlargement are also frequency and urgency, as previously stated. Many times, these symptoms resolve after surgery, but if they do not, you may be treated with medications, biofeedback, or pelvic muscle stimulation as discussed in Chapters Six and Seven.

If you are incontinent after your TURP, your urologist needs to know so that an evaluation can be undertaken to determine the cause or causes of your leakage. Your evaluation will probably include a urinalysis to make sure that you don't have an infection and a cystoscopy to look inside your bladder. During this procedure, your doctor will be able to see if there is a little bit of prostate tissue remaining that is causing the problem. He or she will also inspect the urethra, the external sphincter, and the bladder neck to assess whether these structures have been injured or if excessive scar tissue formed causing narrowing of the channel. Any of these problems could be causing your leakage and may require another surgery, or antibiotics in the case of infection.

If cystoscopy and urinalysis don't reveal the cause of your leakage, a urodynamic evaluation will be done. I often call it a bladder function test, as opposed to the cystoscopy, which tells us what the bladder and the urethra look like. This test gives us insight as to how the bladder is working and is described in Chapter Three. Briefly, a catheter is placed through your urethra into your bladder. This catheter will fill your bladder with fluid and measure the pressures generated by your bladder in response to the filling. Either sticky patches or hair-thin needles will be placed around your perineum (bottom side). These patches will measure the activity of the pelvic muscles. What this test reveals will direct the treatment.

Stress Incontinence

If stress incontinence is the problem and it is due to injury to the external sphincter, it is possible that you will need surgery to correct your problem. Once again, it is worth trying other therapies first. Medications such as phenylpropanolamine, psuedoephedrine, and imipramine may be tried. Biofeedback or pelvic muscle stimulation may also be tried. And if you just can't stomach the thought of another surgery, a device called a Cunningham clamp or a C3 device can be used. These devices are cushioned clamps placed externally around the penis to close the urethra. You will need to monitor the skin carefully when using these devices. They can occlude the blood flow to the penis if applied too tightly, causing skin breakdown and sores. Therefore, these devices must be released every few hours during use to inspect the skin and prevent breakdown. Many patients will wear one of these devices if they are going out or when they are doing activities that cause their leakage.

Prostate Cancer and Surgery

Before I talk about surgeries to treat postprostatectomy incontinence (PPI), I need to talk about surgery for prostate cancer, as the statistics about incontinence after a radical prostatectomy vary and depend on the researcher's definition of incontinence. Some say that people who leak and don't wear pads are continent. It is important before surgery to know as much as possible about your surgeon's own ideas about incontinence. How does the doctor define incontinence? How often has the surgeon performed a radical prostatectomy? What is the surgeon's personal incontinence rate with this surgery? If possible, talk to patients who have had this surgery. We believe that men who learn how to do Kegel exercises before surgery may have a slightly lower rate of incontinence, and those who start Kegel exercises shortly after surgery become dry sooner.

A radical prostatectomy is removal of the entire prostate, as opposed to a TURP, which removes only the portion that is blocking the urethra. The prostate is removed along with a portion of the urethra. The remaining urethra is rejoined to the base of the bladder. The muscles of the internal sphincter are removed, leaving the external sphincter as the only urinary control mechanism. After the surgery, you will have a catheter in place for 7 to 21 days. This allows the surgical area to heal. Once the catheter is removed, it is likely that you will have some degree of incontinence for a short period of time, ranging from total lack of control to occasional dripping. In general, this leakage resolves over 3 to 6 months. If your incontinence continues beyond one year and is bothersome to you, you should be evaluated. This evaluation will be similar to the one done after the TURP, except that your doctor may also be concerned about a cancer recurrence. If it looks as if surgery is the only option to get you dry, you have two choices: a collagen injection or an artificial sphincter.

Collagen Injections

Prior to the injection, a skin test must be performed and the site of the test observed by you for one month to ensure that you are not allergic to the material being used for the procedure (collagen). If there is no reaction, you may proceed with the surgery. Usually, it is done in the hospital operating room under anesthesia, although some urologists are now performing this procedure in the office with local anesthetic. The injection is either through the urethra via the penis or through the bladder via the abdomen. The collagen is injected at the junction of the bladder and the urethra just as it is in women. For the transurethral method, the cystoscope is passed through the penis to the level to be injected. The collagen is then injected until the urethra closes.

The success rate with this procedure has not been too encouraging. It will take more than one injection session to become dry. According to an article from the University of Iowa in the June 1997 issue of *Urology*, only 8 percent of the patients in the study achieved significant improvement, 32 percent had minimal improvement, and 60 percent had no significant improvement. Researchers also found that neither the number of injection procedures nor the volume of material used correlated to success.

A newer way to perform this procedure is to inject the collagen into the bladder neck through the bladder using scopes through the abdomen. While it is hoped that this will increase the continence rates, the long-term statistics are not yet available.

Artificial Sphincter

The artificial sphincter has been the mainstay of therapy for PPI for many years. Placement of the sphincter requires surgery and a stay in the hospital of one to three days. The success rate after placement of the sphincter—that is, no leakage—is approximately 85 to 95 percent, with patient satisfaction with the device actually being a little higher. Over time, the continence rate decreases slightly, probably due to atrophy or shrinkage of the surrounding tissue, malfunction of the sphincter, or loss of fluid in the reservoir. Herein lies the problem with the device: It is artificial and occasionally prone to failure. Also, artificial material increases the risk of infection. If infection occurs, the device must be removed. This risk is highest in the first week or two after surgery. With today's antibiotics, the infection rate is relatively low. Also, as with any mechanical device, there is the risk of malfunction. With the newer devices, again this risk is relatively low.

The sphincter consists of three parts: a reservoir, a pump, and a cuff. The cuff is placed around the urethra and acts as the actual sphincter. The pump is placed in the scrotum and the reservoir is placed near the bladder in the abdomen. There is tubing connecting each of these parts. Immediately after the surgery, the device will be deactivated to allow the urethra to heal prior to applying pressure with the cuff. Your device may remain deactivated for three to six weeks depending on your surgeon's preference. Once your sphincter is activated, some of the fluid from your reservoir is transferred to the cuff, thereby compressing the urethra. When you feel the need to void, you press the pump in your scrotum a few times. This transfers fluid from the cuff back into the reservoir, releasing the compression on the urethra. Urine then flows, the bladder empties, and over the next two minutes the cuff refills, again compressing the urethra. Some urologists like to have the patient deactivate the cuff at night, allowing for increased blood flow to the urethra and decreased risk of cuff erosion, which occurs when the cuff cuts into the urethra. When this happens, the cuff must be removed. Deactivation of the cuff is particularly important if you have had radiation to the pelvis, as the tissues are already damaged from the radiation.

While postprostatectomy incontinence can be devastating, the important things to remember are that it is treatable, there are a variety of treatments to try, and that evaluation of the cause of your leakage is absolutely necessary to provide you with the most appropriate therapy.

TEN

Treatments Available to the Neurologically Challenged

*"Do not let what you cannot do interfere
with what you can do."*
—JOHN WOODEN

For a health care provider, treating people with neurologic problems can be one on the most difficult challenges. Health care providers can only offer people with neurologic problems a management solution, rather than a cure. As in all areas of incontinence, the management solutions are only as good as the skills and knowledge of the provider. Often, people with neurologic diseases either stabilize with significant disability, as in stroke, or continue to lose function over time, as in multiple sclerosis (MS).

Sometimes, the nature of the disorder is somewhat more elusive, as when you have an old back injury or a trauma to your tailbone. In these cases, your bladder problems may have crept up slowly, making it difficult to remember when your problem started. People with back and neck problems often fall into this category. Even though these injuries aren't diseases, there is damage to the nerves. Depending on where in your back your injury is located, different symptoms will appear. Treating bladder problems as a result of these injuries can be difficult. The problems can change over the years, as well as from day to day and even during the course of the day. In addition, medications that are used to treat your disease can cause additional bladder problems.

Mixed Signals

When treating the neurologic diseases, it is helpful to keep in mind that what is happening to your larger leg muscles may also be happening to your pelvic muscles. If your leg is spastic, it is likely that your pelvic muscle is spastic also. If your spasticity is happening only on one side, it will also happen on the same side of your pelvic muscle. This is because your pelvic muscles are controlled by some of the same nerve roots that control your leg muscles. If you have a flaccid leg or weakness on one side, your pelvic muscle will be weak on the same side. In reality, this means that your muscles won't provide added closure when needed. If your pelvic muscles are completely paralyzed, you may not have any closure of the urethra at all, in which case you might experience constant leaking.

Sometimes, in the neurologic diseases, the area of the brain affected may make getting to the bathroom difficult, while at other times the area affected may be responsible for interpreting the signals coming from the bladder. The signals may not only come strongly, but your brain has no ability to discriminate as to whether these are signals that should send you charging to the bathroom or signals that might suggest only keeping your eyes open for the bathroom. Other problems are that the early warning signals may be sent too late, so by the time you get the signal, your bladder is almost at capacity. Other times, the signal just doesn't get through at all.

After a stroke or with MS, the bladder may have to work hard pushing urine out (as when the pelvic muscle is spastic) and it eventually becomes very thickened (hypertrophied). A thickened bladder may be an irritable bladder, sending messages frequently to the brain, making it hard for you to predict when you actually do have a full bladder. The thickness of the bladder causes it to hold a smaller amount of urine and causes the bladder to stretch less. A thick bladder can give a slight squeeze and the strength of the contraction is enough to bypass the sphincter's strength. Another danger is that eventually the pressure becomes so high inside the bladder that urine is pushed back up into the kidneys, which may eventually cause decreased kidney function. If you have this type of bladder, you should be seen routinely by a urologist so that the function of both your bladder and kidneys is monitored on a regular basis. Depending on the bladder pressures found during your evaluation, an indwelling catheter, a straight catheter schedule, or a diversion of the ureters completely away from the bladder might be recommended.

Missed Signals

Another type of neurologic change is that the bladder may not respond to the brain's signals, either because the signals aren't generated or the signals don't get through. With this type of problem, your bladder may become a big, floppy bag that won't contract with enough strength to empty completely. It will keep stretching to fill until you experience pain, which then becomes the signal to go to the toilet, or you become incontinent. When you have this problem, you develop all types of tricks to empty completely, from bending over, to pushing on your belly, to toileting twice in a row. Another trick is to go to the bathroom frequently. You are prone to urinary tract infections because your bladder is never emptied completely. Because urine does not empty completely, you may also have problems with bladder stones. Usually, other than the urinary tract infections and being prone to stones, this problem isn't a big worry to your health care provider if your bladder pressure is low. It is easily resolved using a straight catheter on a regular basis to empty the bladder completely.

The Importance of a Specialist

As you can see, if you have a neurologic disease, you have some very special needs. It would be nice to be able to say that a person with a neurologic disorder has one type of bladder problem; however, most of these problems are mixed in nature, one symptom overlapping another. No matter what the actual bladder problem, however, these needs are treatable if not curable.

It is best if these bladder problems are treated by a specialist. The job of the provider is to prevent damage to your kidneys and then to see if your situation can be improved. Therefore, it is important that you choose a provider who has experience working with patients with neurologic problems. Another thing to keep in mind is that you will probably have the most contact with nurses. It is important that the nursing staff understand and listen so that you can receive the maximum benefit from your doctor. A specialist who will not refer you to outside agencies or providers is not the specialist for you!

Once you find a specialist you like and trust, you have an obligation to stay with the specialist and try the treatments suggested. It is tempting to switch to a doctor who paints a rosier picture, because you want a cure! However, these problems wax and wane but rarely get better. If you have found a specialist who is willing to stick with you through all the management, you must be willing to work at the treatment when things seem to be going well or not so well. The treatment for these problems is never simple and the first treatment is rarely the one and only thing that needs to be done in this situation. If you keep focused on good management and continue to work with your physician, you will find a satisfactory solution!

ELEVEN

Maintaining Continence as You Age

*"Even if you are on the right track, you will get run over
if you just sit there."*
—WILL ROGERS

Like people with neurologic problems, if you are elderly (age 65 or older) you have some special needs when it comes to maintaining continence. By the very nature of your age, you have had multiple insults over the years to your back, abdomen, and pelvic muscles. In addition, your organ function begins to decline, nerve and muscle changes take place, and the ability to receive messages from sensory nerves and organs diminishes. All this adds up to a pretty large incontinence risk. As you age, your bladder changes in several ways. Whether these changes are the result of a lifetime of wear and tear, disease processes, or medications is unknown at this time. We do know that as people age their bladder becomes less stretchable, holds less volume, and becomes more irritable, which leads to increased frequency, nighttime toileting, and occasionally leaking on the way to the bathroom.

Alzheimer's and Parkinson's Diseases

Diseases such as Alzheimer's and Parkinson's affect the bladder and your ability to interpret signals sent from your bladder. In Parkinson's disease, your pelvic muscles become increasingly spastic, which causes your bladder to work harder to empty against a "closed door." As your bladder becomes more muscular, it becomes thicker and less and less stretchable. It also becomes more irritable. Therefore, you feel the urge to go to the bathroom frequently and when you get there you cannot initiate a stream because your pelvic muscle won't relax. Coupled with this frustrating situation is the problem that many Parkinson's patients suffer from a hesitancy in their walking and an intention tremor. Getting to the bathroom within the two-minute warning period is going to be difficult at best. If you get there, getting your clothes unzipped is tough because of the shakiness of your hands. The inability to empty often leads to small volume voiding and around-the-clock leaking. Your problem is best managed by periodically emptying your bladder throughout the day or using an indwelling catheter if the problem is severe.

If you care for a person with Alzheimer's disease, you have a unique situation because the progressive loss of memory may eventually lead to leaking around the clock. However, the mechanism of leaking is slightly different than in the Parkinson's patient. With Alzheimer's disease, the patient can no longer interpret the signals that the bladder is sending, so the urge to toilet is ignored until it is too late. When the patient is full, he or she often feels pain and becomes restless and combative, making it difficult for the attendant to get the patient to the bathroom before leaking. As the disease progresses, the patient can no longer find the toilet and later doesn't understand what the toilet is used for. This is frustrating to the caregiver and sometimes leads to abuse of these patients. The best option early in the disease is to gently remind the patient when to toilet and lead him or her there. As the patient becomes increasingly forgetful, the caregiver may need to institute a two-hour toileting schedule around the clock so that the patient does not become restless and combative. At this point, the caregiver may need to gently place the patient on the toilet and run water to help the patient start the process of voiding. As the disease progresses, often the only option is a diaper or an indwelling catheter.

Age-Related Changes

Aside from Alzheimer's and Parkinson's patients, treating the elderly is often a matter of increasing the bladder capacity, strengthening the external sphincter (the pelvic or Kegel) muscles, and changing some bad habits that have developed over time. Treating the bad habits is usually the first line of defense. Like all incontinent people, you should avoid bladder irritants such as excessive citrus fruit intake (including juices), caffeine, and aspartame. Because of leaking on the way to the bathroom caused by both your irritable bladder and decreased capacity, you tend to get into the habit of going to the bathroom frequently. As we have learned, an irritable bladder is an irritable bladder no matter how much it holds. Toileting frequently won't change the number of times you leak, only the amount. The trick is to train your bladder into holding more urine and asking it to settle down. You need strong pelvic muscles. The good news is that in the elderly a little strength goes a long way, because activity is usually less than in a younger group of people.

Using Kegel exercises to inhibit your bladder and strengthen the pelvic muscles as discussed in Chapter Seven is the most important thing you can do to help your bladder to become more normal. Doing 5 to 10 Kegel exercises two to three times a day is usually enough to help you regain control. If you are having trouble doing Kegel contractions, see a health provider for an examination as you attempt the exercises. A health provider will also evaluate the condition of the vagina or rectum and make a determination as to whether you would be a candidate for pelvic muscle stimulation (Chapter Seven). A health provider can help you evaluate what you are doing wrong and you will begin to see rapid improvement within a short time.

Another problem for you may be getting to the bathroom quickly, especially after you are awakened with the urge to void. By the time you sit up, dangle your legs at the bedside, and get those creaky knees and hips moving, it may be too late! Really look at your surroundings and try to determine if there is a way to bring the toilet closer to you. Maybe changing to a closer bedroom or using a commode or urinal is all that's needed.

If you have heart problems, the heart pumps more efficiently when you lie down, so even if you have no problems during the day you might have trouble with frequent toileting at night because the kidneys are processing all the fluid that your heart is busily pumping to them. It may help to elevate your legs above the level of your heart for 30 to 45 minutes right before bedtime. This in effect fools your kidneys into processing the increased fluid before you go to sleep. After elevating your legs, go to the bathroom before you go to sleep and then see if you don't get just a few more hours of sleep at a time.

If you take a diuretic to help get rid of extra fluid, you are tied to the bathroom for an hour every day after you take your water pill. Unfortunately, there is not much you can do other than grin and bear it. With your health care provider's permission, possibly the dose of the pill could be divided to make the diuresis less dramatic at any one time. Make sure these pills are taken before 4 P.M. so that you are not running to the bathroom all night.

One of the easiest things you can do if you are a woman is replace the moisture and improve the vaginal skin's integrity with estrogen cream or a vaginal moisturizer such as Replens (see Chapter Six). Vaginally delivered estrogen is usually quite safe for the elderly, is better tolerated than the oral preparation, and does not lead to breakthrough bleeding or spotting as oral preparations can in this age group. Estrogen improves blood flow to the mucosa, plumps up the tissue, and increases lubrication. In theory, this should help close the urethra, but this has not been proven. What we do know from clinical experience is that estrogen seems to improve problems with urgency, which makes sense when you consider that the urethra is derived from the same tissue as the vagina and has almost as many estrogen receptors. While vaginal moisturizers do not work in the same fashion as estrogen, they do discourage dryness and improve vaginal comfort. When the vaginal tissue is in good shape, the likelihood of infection decreases. Less vaginal infections mean less bladder infections. Estrogen cream is also an important tool in the use of pessaries (see Chapter Six). The combination of estrogen cream and pessary use has improved many elderly women's incontinence with a minimum of fuss.

TWELVE

Dysfunctional Voiding

"Insanity is doing the same things over and over again,
but expecting different results."
—Rita Mae Brown

We alluded to dysfunctional voiding in Chapter Two when talking about problems people have when they are unable to empty their bladder completely. Although no two groups agree on the definition of dysfunctional or on the constellation of symptoms, it is generally recognized that this problem is due to the inability to relax the pelvic muscles enough to empty the bladder in an efficient manner. Some clinicians call this problem *pseudodysynergia*. Urologists see this problem in men and often diagnose it as chronic prostatitis. Gynecologists may call the same symptoms in women vaginismus, while physical therapists might recognize it as trigger points or a spastic pelvic muscle. Clinicians used to feel vaginismus, pseudodysynergia, or a spastic pelvic muscle were "junk" diagnoses because we couldn't define the problem. However, as more and more clinicians become proficient at urodynamic testing, they are recognizing this syndrome for the problem that it is.

Causes

Dysfunctional voiding can be characterized as secondary to a preexisting problem. Usually, the root causes are in one of three areas: most commonly in the neurologic system or musculoskeletal systems, or less commonly a psychological problem.

Neurologic causes of dysfunctional voiding happen because the nerves telling the muscles to relax are no longer intact, or sensation to the pelvic area is lacking. This can be the result of a neurologic disease such as multiple sclerosis, or congenital spinal cord defects such as spina bifida or spinal cord injury. Essentially, the muscles are capable of working efficiently, but the message from the brain is garbled.

If the cause is musculoskeletal, the muscles themselves are in spasm. Often, this is related to a neurologic problem, but not always. After abdominal or pelvic surgery or accidents involving the trunk of your body, scar tissue (adhesions) sometimes forms around the organs near the site of this damage. Like scars on your skin, this tissue doesn't stretch or move like the surrounding tissue. In some cases, the scar tissue is so extensive that it shows up on testing done with ultrasound or magnetic resonance imaging (MRI). The scar tissue formation usually isn't a problem. Normally it will stretch during daily activities. However, if the tissue doesn't stretch or binds some of the internal organs, you can have symptoms caused by that binding. Organs such as the colon or bladder may have trouble stretching to accommodate their contents and thus produce urgency, and in severe cases, pain. If the scar tissue is in the connective tissue that lines your body's cavities or envelops the muscles (fascia), it can cause the muscles to function improperly. Although how this happens is poorly understood, it is thought that the scar tissue pulls the skeleton out of alignment. The lower back and hips rotate as a result. This pulls on the connections of the muscles to the skeleton, causing pain and spasm of the muscles. In severe cases, the nerves coming out of the spinal cord can be compressed as the spinal column twists. This may cause numbness and tingling or even lack of sensation to the legs and pelvic area.

Finally, there is a lot of controversy surrounding the causes that are considered psychological in nature. Many clinicians feel that people who were raped or sexually traumatized are more prone to this problem. Indeed, some studies have found that there is a slightly higher rate of dysfunctional voiding in this population, but the problem doesn't exist at the level formerly believed. When the condition exists because of this kind of trauma, it should be treated using a combination of therapies, including counseling. Trauma will often cause people to protect the hurt area by guarding it and tightening up the muscles. Just the expectation of pain or the memory of a painful time can cause a person to subconsciously tighten those muscles. This situation can also occur after bad urinary tract or vaginal infections.

Symptoms

People who have voiding dysfunction may experience a variety of symptoms. Some have urinary frequency, difficulty emptying their bladder completely, or a stream of urine sounds different or interrupted compared to other people's streams. Sometimes they have incontinence that consists of a few drops or a continuously small amount of leaking. Sometimes it hurts to urinate and intercourse can be painful. Often, patients will complain of pain in and around the vagina, or the tip of the penis, into the scrotum, and near their anus and tailbone. On examination, no infection of either the urinary tract or vagina can be found. Almost always, the urodynamic test is normal or shows a small capacity or early sensation. It is easy to see why this problem is so difficult to recognize and why it has so many names. The definitive study for this problem is an electromyelogram (EMG) of the pelvic muscles performed during the urodynamic testing. Using skin patches (needles cause pain and may mask the problem), the technician studies the EMG tracings throughout the filling and voiding phases of the study. In patients with this problem, the EMG tracings are of a higher amplitude and are more erratic during the filling phase and inappropriately elevated during the voiding study. This result indicates that pelvic muscles are not functioning properly. It takes a skilled urodynamicist to recognize and interpret these patterns.

The elevation of EMG tracings during the voiding phase of the study is particularly meaningful. When the patient's bladder has to empty against a pelvic muscle that has not relaxed when voiding, the bladder must push harder. It is similar to trying to void when the pelvic muscle is slammed shut. The bladder pushes harder to compensate for the pelvic muscle not opening when it should to let the urine out. The bladder eventually builds up more strength by building more muscle (much like when you pump iron). The walls of the bladder become thicker, less stretchable, and often more irritable. In worst-case scenarios, you can't empty completely, which can cause urinary tract infections and/or reflux of urine back up into the kidneys. Although the cure may be simple—relaxing the pelvic muscles—the treatment is complex.

Treatments

Some of you who have had this problem in the past may have been treated with urethral dilatation or stretching of the urethral muscle. Although reportedly effective in the short term, in the long term this treatment may cause permanent damage to the sphincter or urethra.

Today, there are several treatments, although it may take your provider some trial and error to discover the etiology of the problem and to find a treatment that works for you. Obviously, the first thing is to get an excellent history and physical including a sexual history and palpation of the pelvic muscles, vagina, and rectum for tender spots. A good urodynamic exam including an EMG must be done and it may be helpful to have cystoscopy (look into the bladder) to determine the condition of the bladder wall. Once the diagnosis is made and a cause is attributed, the treatment of this problem varies considerably from provider to provider.

Much of the treatment chosen will depend on the resources available. Many times, treatment starts with the use of a muscle relaxant. Occasionally, a tricyclic antidepressant will be used to increase the threshold for pain. Soothing topical agents may be used to treat pain. Warm baths and perineal massage (also used in preparing the vaginal muscles for childbirth) will frequently be prescribed to relax the pelvic muscles. If the provider knows of a biofeedback therapist, you will likely be referred for therapy. The purpose is to help you identify your pelvic muscles and to teach you to use them appropriately. It also helps to strengthen these muscles, since tired and weak muscles are more prone to spasm. In cases where the patient has a great deal of difficulty identifying the muscle to relax, pelvic muscle stimulation can be used. Essentially, the provider is working in a backward fashion by strengthening the muscle enough so that you can learn the difference between contracting and relaxing. Pelvic muscle stimulation provides another benefit in that it blocks the painful impulses from the spasm. In cases where scar tissue formation is suspected, a referral to physical therapy is appropriate. Physical therapists who know how to do myofascial and trigger-point release therapies are crucial in this situation. They will gently work the tissue over time in order to stretch it and restore mobility. This frees up the joints and the organs that have been banded by the tissue. Often, this treatment eliminates the problem.

Physical therapists will also work to strengthen the surrounding muscles so that they can help support the work of the damaged muscles. In cases of suspected nerve impingement, an MRI of the spine and tailbone areas should be done and the appropriate referrals made if there is an abnormality. It is not at all unusual to see a combination of these treatments prescribed in an effort to find something that works for you. Be patient: Often a management program takes a while to implement and even longer to see results. Throughout treatment it is very important to stay in contact with your health care provider about what works and what doesn't.

THIRTEEN

Children and Incontinence

"Success breeds confidence."
—BERYL MARKHAM

How Children Learn Continence

Generally, a child has developed enough to begin learning "proper" toileting around age 2. A few learn a little earlier and many a little later. Remember, the bladder's job in life is to store and get rid of urine, and at age 2, a child's nervous system may have developed enough to begin to intervene in this filling and emptying cycle. The child can then learn to stop the bladder from emptying whenever it wants and that glorious day arrives when diapers can be thrown away.

Most children are able to control their bladder the majority of the time between ages 2 and 3. The most vexing problem for many parents is the child who continues to wet the bed. It is known that a child whose parents were bedwetters has a 70 percent chance of having this difficulty, and that bedwetting is more common in boys than in girls. Bedwetting occurs in 15 percent of 5-year-olds, 5 percent of 10-year-olds, and 1 percent of 15-year-olds.

There are many reasons for bedwetting, also called nocturnal enuresis. As stated previously, if the parents were bedwetters, the children are more likely to have this problem. Delay of maturation of the nervous system is also speculated to be a cause, as are food allergies, though no particular food can be implicated. For children who were initially dry at night, chronic illness, parental separation, a new sibling, or other such stressors have been implicated.

Diagnosing Bedwetting

Treatment for bedwetting is often undertaken once a child is old enough to want to have sleepovers. A careful history is taken to be sure that there are no daytime problems. If there is no difficulty at any other time, if the physical examination is normal, and if the urine test for bacteria is negative, no other test may be performed and treatment is initiated. When a child has day- and night-control problems, such as frequency, urgency, and/or incontinence, and these symptoms occur regularly, more evaluation will likely be needed. The doctor will talk to you and your child about the nature of the problem, so be prepared to be specific about when the problem occurs, for example, she might have control problems only when she laughs. You will also be asked about your child's bowel habits, whether the problem is new, and possibly about anything that may have happened while you were pregnant. The doctor will examine your child, including looking at the position of the urethra, examining the anus, and looking at his back. Tests may be performed. The test you can count on is a urinalysis, so make sure your child knows she may need to urinate in a cup. If the urine test is negative, the doctor may refer your child to a specialist or order X-rays to look at the urinary tract.

The most common X-rays for these problems are an intravenous pyelogram or IVP, a voiding cystourethrogram or VCUG, and a renal ultrasound. If you are seeing a specialist, a urodynamic evaluation may be ordered (see Chapter Five). The purpose of these tests is to make sure that there is no abnormality in your child's urinary tract and to assess whether there may be a neurologic problem. The findings of these tests will determine the ultimate treatment. These tests are important because abnormalities could cause long-term damage to the kidneys.

Treatments for Bedwetting

There are a variety of options available and all will usually include decreasing the amount of liquid taken just before bed. It is recommended that bladder irritants be decreased, such as soda and caffeinated drinks, especially in the late afternoon and evening. Children should stop all liquid intake approximately two hours before bed. If this regimen does not stop the problem, then bedwetting alarms may be tried. These devices will attempt to awaken the child as he begins to wet. Eventually, it is hoped that with these alarms the child will begin to wake up on his own prior to the initiation of the void. If these suggestions are of no benefit, medications may be tried.

The medications that are used to treat nocturnal enuresis are the same as those used to treat urge incontinence in adults, oxybutynin and imipramine, which were discussed in Chapter Six. An additional medication, DDAVP (desmopressin acetate), is used specifically for bedwetting. DDAVP is similar to a hormone that is made naturally by all of us, and it acts to decrease the amount of urine that is produced. It is available as a nasal spray and as a tablet. It is successful in decreasing bedwetting episodes in 70 percent of children, according to many studies.

The most important thing for you to remember if you have a child who is a bedwetter is that while it is frustrating for both you and your child, most children do not have a physical abnormality and will eventually achieve complete bladder control. Remember that children develop at different rates, and the large majority have achieved "normal" adult voiding habits by age 5. If you believe your child has a problem, speak with his or her pediatrician as soon as possible so that kidney damage can be avoided.

FOURTEEN

Interstitial Cystitis

"An unspoken expectation is an impossible expectation."
—KATHY PEEL

Interstitial cystitis is a painful, often debilitating, disease of the bladder. The symptoms are severe frequency, urgency, and pain in the lower abdomen or perineum that are relieved with urination. To get an idea of what this feels like, think of being on a long car trip in the middle of nowhere after just drinking a thermos of coffee. A road sign says that the next rest room is 25 miles away. Think of how desperate you will feel by the time you get to that rest stop. Now, think of feeling that way all the time. This may be interstitial cystitis.

Diagnosis

Interstitial cystitis is more likely to be diagnosed in women, although men with the diagnosis of chronic prostatitis may also have this disease. The median age of onset is 40 years. It is more common in whites than blacks, and much more common in those of Jewish descent. The cause of this disease is unknown. There is much speculation and research, with autoimmune illness and allergic reactions as possible causes.

Many times, you will be referred to a specialist by your family doctor if you have been diagnosed with recurrent urinary tract infections, especially if it takes more than one course of antibiotics to cure your symptoms. It is important that you bring your urine test results with you to your first appointment. The doctor will ask you about the onset of symptoms, whether you can associate any particular activity with the onset of symptoms (for example, sex), or if anything you eat or drink worsens your symptoms. You will be asked how long it takes for your symptoms to resolve if you have been treated with antibiotics. If you are not having symptoms at the time of your visit, and your physical exam is normal (which it often is), you may be asked to return when you are symptomatic. This is to assure that your symptoms are not related to vaginal infection, abnormal urinalysis (infection), or pelvic muscle dysfunction. Often, your doctor will ask you to complete a voiding diary with and without symptoms. The average patient with interstitial cystitis will void approximately 16 times per day, volumes with each void averaging 75 milliliters, which is a little more than a quarter cup of urine. Don't forget that the normal volume with each void is between one and two cups of urine, with a frequency of every two to four hours depending on fluid intake.

There are other tests that can be done to help with the diagnosis; they are not always necessary and often treatment is begun based on symptoms with normal urinalysis. One of the most common tests is a cystoscopy. The doctor looks in your bladder with a scope inserted into the bladder through the urethra. This test will often be conducted in the hospital while you are under an anesthetic. Stretching of the bladder (called hydrodistention) is done at the same time. Anesthetics are given because hydrodistention is painful if done while you are awake. The doctor is checking your bladder capacity and your bladder lining. Frequently, the bladder lining of a person with interstitial cystitis will crack and bleed with overstretching, but this can also happen in people without bladder symptoms. Your bladder capacity under anesthesia will usually be significantly less than 1,000 milliliters or 5 cups if you have interstitial cystitis, but you can have the disease and have a normal bladder capacity. Approximately 50 percent of the time, this test can also decrease symptoms, with some people experiencing long-term relief. Immediately after the procedure, your symptoms may become worse, lasting up to one month. Your symptoms worsen because your bladder lining is damaged further with the hydrodistension (overstretching). It is believed that improvement occurs once the lining has healed. Just remember that this is actually a good sign, because many will have long-lasting relief from this procedure. Also during your procedure, your doctor may do biopsies of your bladder to make sure that you do not have cancer, although cancer is very unlikely. A Hunner's ulcer may also be discovered. If it is seen, it almost always means you have interstitial cystitis. This is not an ulcer like those found in the stomach, but is a red patch that looks very suspicious for cancer, so if one is found you can be sure that your bladder will be biopsied (a piece of tissue sent to the laboratory for analysis). These ulcers are not commonly seen.

Another newer test that is done is called the potassium chloride test. It will indicate if the lining of your bladder is normal, which it will not be if you have interstitial cystitis. Your doctor will place two solutions in your bladder using a catheter. One solution will be plain water, a small amount of which will be put into your bladder. Your doctor will then ask whether this has worsened your symptoms. The water will then be drained. Next, a small amount of potassium chloride will be put into your bladder. In 70 percent of people with interstitial cystitis, the symptoms will worsen. You should feel better once the solution is washed from your bladder. Of course, your doctor may try to fool you and put the potassium solution in your bladder first.

Theories About the Cause of Interstitial Cystitis

One of the theories of the disease is that the lining of the bladder (the glycosaminoglycan [GAG] layer) has been injured by some unknown insult, which causes it to become leaky—that is, to allow the nerves of the bladder to "see" substances that they are not meant to see. The nerves become "revved up," which leads to pain. Before the nerves are revved up, the bladder responds in the only way it knows, causing frequency and urgency.

Treatments

With the finding that the lining of the bladder is damaged has come the first drug marketed specifically for this disease, Elmiron or pentosanpolysulfate. This drug helps bladder surface defense mechanisms to detoxify agents in the urine. Elmiron is taken three times per day. The tablets are 100 milligrams. It may take three to six months before there is any change in your symptoms. In the meantime, there are other treatments that can be used.

Dimethylsulfoxide (DMSO) has been used to treat interstitial cystitis for many years. This medication is placed into the bladder on a weekly basis, usually for six to eight weeks, through a temporary catheter inserted in the bladder at the doctor's office. If there has been a significant change in your symptoms, you should continue with a maintenance dose of one treatment per month. Often this medication is used in conjunction with others in the form of a "cocktail." The other medications that are frequently used are heparin, steroids, and lidocaine.

Heparin helps replace the GAG layer that is believed to be destroyed, steroids may help with the inflammatory response that is sometimes seen, and lidocaine helps numb the bladder. There are no significant side effects of DMSO in humans. Most patients and their families complain of a strong garlic odor the first day or two after a treatment. DMSO has been associated with cataracts in animals, so it is recommended that you have an eye exam every three to six months if you are on chronic therapy.

Other medications can be placed into the bladder in an effort to relieve symptoms. They are silver nitrate and sodium oxychlorosene or Chlorpactin WCS-90. Often, these medications will be placed while you are under an anesthetic. Antidepressants are also used in the treatment of this disease. The most common is amitriptyline. This medication is given at bedtime in doses ranging from 10 to 75 milligrams. It has a sedative effect (makes you sleepy) and may increase your tolerance to pain. Other antidepressants that can be prescribed are Prozac and Zoloft. All of these antidepressants make this disease easier to live with, since people who suffer with chronic pain are usually depressed.

Because of the belief that there may be an allergic component to interstitial cystitis, often antihistamines are used in addition to some of the other treatments mentioned. Antihistamines are the drugs you might take in the spring when you have an allergic reaction to pollen with itchy, watery eyes and sneezing. For some IC patients, spring is the worst time for their bladder symptoms. Medications such as diphenhydramine (Benadryl) or hydroxyzine (Atarax) and (Vistaril) may relieve your symptoms. The main side effect of these medications can be drowsiness or dry mouth.

Infrequently, surgery is performed to treat IC. Attempts to disable the nerves to the bladder have been tried and so far have not been very effective. Bladder augmentation, or enlarging the bladder, has also been done, but has not been found to be effective, because the bladder is not truly small; it only seems to be for the patient with this disease. Removal of the bladder and diversion of the urine has been the most successful surgery. It is a major operation and is reserved for people who have not had success with other forms of therapy.

A newer procedure is being performed, which is the implantation of a nerve stimulator into the lower part of the spinal column. This procedure was described in Chapter Eight. It is not specifically approved for interstitial cystitis, but is approved for the treatment of urgency and urge incontinence. Patients have also found relief from TENS units (external nerve stimulators), pelvic muscle stimulation, and acupuncture.

Although interstitial cystitis (IC) is a disease of the bladder lining, so far we know little about the causes of the disease, treatments that consistently work, or how to prevent the disease from occurring in the first place. If you have a diagnosis of interstitial cystitis, your disease is presently considered a chronic condition. Although we don't yet have a cure for the disease, we do have many treatment strategies. Often, you and your physician may need to try several strategies before finding one that works for you. Therefore, it is extremely important that you seek a second opinion before considering treatments that effect a permanent change in the way your body functions and also that you communicate regularly with your physician. We hope that soon a cure and prevention strategy will be found for this disease. Until then, knowledge about your disease is your best weapon.

POSTSCRIPT

"Think of it as being easy, and it shall be easy. Think of it
as being difficult, and it shall be difficult."
—ARABIAN PROVERB

We have attempted to educate you on the pervasive problem of urinary incontinence and to let you know that you do not have to suffer
with this problem. As you have seen, many of the treatments require
a commitment of work from you, such as biofeedback and pelvic
muscle stimulation, in order to be successful. However, these treatments do not have side effects or significant complications. Surgeries, on the other hand, require you to follow the instructions of
your physician regarding postoperative care, have the risk of failing
over time, and can have significant complications and side effects.
Surgery can render you dry quickly, as opposed to biofeedback and
pelvic muscle stimulation, which can take weeks to correct your
problem and a lifetime of exercises to remain successful. In general,
it is up to you how you proceed, but we hope you think carefully
about the options and are now armed with the knowledge to make
good choices about your care. It is our hope that you live a long,
happy, and dry life!

"Let me remember that each life must follow its own
course, and that what happens to other people has
absolutely nothing to do with what happens to me."
—MARJORIE HOLMES

GLOSSARY

Alzheimer's disease   A progressive neurologic disease characterized by increasing forgetfulness, labile emotions, and poor judgment.

Artificial urinary sphincter   A mechanical device surgically implanted in the patient to control the opening and closing of the urethra manually.

Behavioral techniques   Specific interventions designed to alter the relationship between the patient's symptoms and his or her environment for the treatment of irregular voiding patterns.

Biofeedback   A behavioral technique through which information about a normally unconscious physiologic process is presented to the patient and the therapist as a visual, auditory, or tactile signal.

Bladder   A distensible muscular organ that stores urine until it is released by the body.

Bladder augmentation   A surgical procedure by which the capacity of the bladder is increased by attaching additional tissue to the bladder.

Bladder-neck prosthesis   A device inserted into a woman's vagina to elevate the bladder neck to the proper position in order to prevent or lessen incontinence.

Bladder-neck suspension   A term for several surgical procedures employed to treat urethral hypermobility.

Bladder training   A behavioral technique that requires the patient to resist or inhibit the sensation of urgency in order to postpone the urge to void.

Catheter   A tube inserted into the body through the urethra or abdomen to allow for urine drainage.

Codes   Numbers assigned to specific disease treatments and types of office visits used by providers to bill their services to insurance companies.

Conservative treatment   Any nonsurgical technique used to treat voiding problems.

Constipation   Difficult or infrequent evacuation of the bowels.

Continence ring   A device inserted into the woman's vagina that provides pressure against the urethra, therefore increasing closure of the urethra.

Copay   A payment that the patient is responsible for when visiting the health care providers.

Cystitis   Inflammation of the bladder.

Cystometrogram (CMG)   A test of the bladder's function that measures the pressure/volume relationship of the bladder to determine the bladder's activity, capacity, sensation, and compliance.

Cystoscopy   A procedure using a scope inserted into the bladder that provides a direct view of the bladder wall.

Detrusor   The smooth muscle in the wall of the bladder that contracts the bladder to expel urine.

Detrusor instability or overactive bladder   An involuntary contraction of the detrusor in the absence of a neurologic disorder.

Detrusor sphincter dyssynergia (DSD)   An inappropriate contraction of the external sphincter occurring at the same time as a contraction of the detrusor.

Diabetes mellitus   A chronic disease of pancreatic origin characterized by insulin deficiency, the inability to utilize carbohydrates, and excess sugar in the blood and urine.

Electrical stimulation   The application of an electrical current to stimulate a muscle contraction or inhibit the nerve supply to the organ being treated.

Electromyelogram (EMG)   The reading of electrical changes generated by contraction of the pelvic muscles.

Fascia   Fibrous tissue laid out in sheets beneath the surface of the skin enveloping the body, enclosing muscles and muscular groups, and separating muscular layers.

Functional incontinence   Urinary incontinence related to the inability to make it to the bathroom in a timely manner because of mobility problems.

Hypertrophy   Enlargement of the bladder muscle usually due to its contracting against a partial obstruction over time.

Intrinsic sphincter deficiency (ISD)   A cause of stress urinary incontinence in which the urethral sphincter is unable to contract and generate sufficient resistance against bladder pressure, usually during maneuvers that increase abdominal pressures (such as coughing, lifting, etc.).

Kidneys   A pair of organs that help to maintain the proper water balance, regulate the acid-base concentration, and process and excrete metabolic wastes.

Mixed incontinence   More than one type of incontinence occurring in the same individual.

Multiple sclerosis (MS)   A degenerative disease of the nervous system in which a hardening of tissue occurs throughout the brain and in the spinal cord.

Overactive bladder   *See **detrusor instability**.*

Overflow incontinence   The involuntary loss of urine associated with the overfilling of the bladder.

Parkinson's disease   A progressive nervous system disease that is characterized by muscular tremor, slowing of movement, facial paralysis, oddity of gait and posture, and weakness.

Pelvic muscle exercises (Kegel contractions)   A technique that requires repetitive active exercise of the pubococcygeus muscle to improve urethral resistance and urinary control.

Pelvic muscle weights   Small weights inserted into the vagina to provide resistance against which the pelvic muscles contract.

Pelvic prolapse   A condition in which the pelvic muscles no longer support the organs of the pelvic cavity.

Periurethral bulking agents   A surgical treatment for urethral insufficiency that involves injecting materials into the periurethral area to increase closure.

Pessary   A device inserted into a woman's vagina in order to increase the support of the pelvic contents.

Postvoid residual volume   The amount of urine left in the bladder immediately following urination.

Preauthorization   A request made to an insurance company to pay for a device or a visit that is normally not covered under the plan in advance of the visit.

Referral   A letter from a provider to another provider requesting care for a patient or a letter from an insurance company granting permission for a patient to see a provider normally not covered by insurance.

Sacral nerve stimulation   A surgical procedure that implants a pacemaking device near the spinal cord. Used to treat severe frequency and urgency.

Sensory urgency   Urgency associated with bladder hypersensitivity.

Sling procedure   A surgical method for treating stress urinary incontinence involving the placement of a sling under the bladder neck.

Stress incontinence   Urinary incontinence characterized by the involuntary loss of urine through the urethra during physical exertion.

Suprapubic tube   A tube inserted surgically through the abdominal wall into the bladder to drain urine from the bladder.

Sutures   Surgical stitches.

Ureters   Thin muscular tubes connecting the kidneys to the bladder.

Urethra   A muscular tube that drains urine from the bladder to the outside of the body.

Urge incontinence   The unintentional loss of urine connected with an abrupt and strong desire to void.

Urge/Urgency   A strong desire to void.

Urinary incontinence   An involuntary loss of urine sufficient to be a problem.

Urinary tract   All of the organs involved in the making, storage, and passage of urine: kidneys, ureters, bladder, and urethra.

Urinary tract infection   An infection in the urinary tract caused by microorganisms.

Urodynamic testing   Tests designed to determine the functioning of the bladder and urethra.

Voiding (or Bladder) Diary   A record of the frequency, timing, amount of voiding, and other factors associated with urinary incontinence.

REFERENCES

Badlani GH. Urologic implications of MS, diabetes, and Parkinson's disease lecture. Fourth National Multi-Specialty Nursing Conference on Urinary Continence, Orlando, Florida, 1998.

Chiarelli, P. *Women's Waterworks Curing Incontinence*. Princeton, NJ: Lewis Lawmen Publishing, Inc., 1992.

Chohan N. *Nursing Drug Handbook*. Springhouse, Pennsylvania: Springhouse Corporation, 1998.

Creasey GH. Electrical stimulation of sacral roots for micturition after spinal cord injury. *Urologic Clinics of North America* 1993;20:505–515.

Dijkema HE, Weil EHJ, Mijs PT, Janknegt RA. Neuromodulation of sacral nerves for incontinence and voiding dysfunction. *European Urology* 1993;24:72–76.

Elbadawi A. Pathology and pathophysiology of detrusor in incontinence. *Urologic Clinics of North America* 1995;22:499–512.

Fantl JA, Newman DK, Colling J, et al. *Managing Acute and Chronic Urinary Incontinence. Clinical Practice Guideline*. Quick Reference Guide for Clinicians, No. 2, 1996 update. Rockville, MD: U.S. Department of Health and Human Services, Public Health Service, Agency for Health Care Policy and Research. AHCPR Pub. No. 96-0686. March 1996.

Foster S. *Herbs for Your Health*. Loveland, CO: Interweave Press, 1996.

Gray M. *Genitourinary Disorders*. St. Louis: Mosby Year Book, Inc., 1992.

Griebling TL, Kreder KJ, Williams RD. Transurethral collagen injection for treatment of postprostatectomy urinary incontinence in men. *Urology* 1997;907–912.

Herman H, Shelly E. Gynecological physical therapy seminar. Memorial Hospital West Fitness and Rehabilitation Center, November 10–12, 1995, Pembroke Pines, Florida.

Himsl KK, Hurwitz, RS. Pediatric urinary incontinence. *Urologic Clinics of North America* 1991;18:283–292.

Holtgrewe HL. Current trends in management of men with lower urinary tract symptoms and benign prostatic hypertrophy. *Urology* supplement to April 1998;1–7.

Ishigooka M, Hashimoto T, Sasagawa I, et al. Electrical pelvic floor stimulation by percutaneous implantable electrode. *British Journal of Urology* 1994;74:191–194.

Klutke JJ, Bergman A. Hormonal influence on the urinary tract. *Urologic Clinics of North America* 1995;22:629–639.

Leach GE, Dmochowski RR, Appell RA, Blaivas JG, Hadley HR, Luber KM, Mostwin JL, O'Donnell PD, Roehrborn CG. Female stress urinary incontinence clinical guidelines panel summary report on surgical management of female stress urinary incontinence. The American Urological Association. *Journal of Urology* 1997;158 (3, Pt. 1):875–880.

McDash Dille C, Kirchhoff KT. Decontamination of vinyl urinary drainage bags with bleach. *Rehabilitation Nursing* 1993;18:292–295.

McGuire EJ, Gudziak MR. *Handbook of Urodynamic Testing.* Covington, GA: Bard Urological Division, 1994.

National Institutes of Health Consensus Development Conference Statement. *Urinary Incontinence in Adults.* U.S. Department of Health and Human Services, 1988;7:1–11.

Rivas DA, Chancellor MB. Neurogenic vesical dysfunction. *Urologic Clinics of North America* 1995;22:579–590.

Sand PK, Richardson DA, Staskin DR, et al. Pelvic floor electrical stimulation in the treatment of genuine stress incontinence: a multicenter, placebo-controlled trial. *American Journal of Obstetrics and Gynecology* 1995;175:72–79.

Schapiro RT, Baumhefner RW, Tourtellotte WW. Multiple sclerosis: a clinical viewpoint to management. *Multiple Sclerosis: Clinical and Pathogenetic Basis.* London: Chapman and Hall, 1997.

Snyder JA, Lipsitz DU. Evaluation of female urinary incontinence. *Urologic Clinics of North America* 1991;18:187–209.

Strange CJ. Incontinence can be controlled. *FDA Consumer. U.S. Food and Drug Administration* 1997;5:28–31.

Wein AJ. Practical uropharmacology. *Urologic Clinics of North America* 1991;18:269–281.

Wein AJ. Pharmacology of incontinence. *Urologic Clinics of North America* 1995;22:557–575.

INDEX